MUSCULAR SYSTEM - ANATOMY, FUNCTIONS AND INJURIES

COMPARTMENT SYNDROME

MEDICAL CAUSES, SYMPTOMS AND SURGICAL OUTCOMES

MUSCULAR SYSTEM - ANATOMY, FUNCTIONS AND INJURIES

Additional books in this series can be found on Nova's website under the Series tab.

Additional e-books in this series can be found on Nova's website under the e-book tab.

MUSCULAR SYSTEM - ANATOMY, FUNCTIONS AND INJURIES

COMPARTMENT SYNDROME

MEDICAL CAUSES, SYMPTOMS AND SURGICAL OUTCOMES

ANNA P. HENDERSON
EDITOR

New York

Library of Congress Cataloging-in-Publication Data

ISBN: 978-1-63482-831-4
Library of Congress Control Number: 2015939093

Published by Nova Science Publishers, Inc. † New York

Contents

Preface

There are various underlying causes which initiate the sequence of events resulting in compartment syndrome including fractures, bleeding, tightly applied casts or extrinsic compressions devices, burns or vigorous exercise. The first chapter of this book serves to review the current understanding of ACS's pathophysiology and highlight implications for the modernization of diagnosis and treatment. The second chapter reviews the evidence relevant to how anesthesiologists can influence the genesis of compartment syndrome. Anesthesia may influence the development of CS through the use of regional anesthesia, optimum blood pressure control and oxygen delivery, and tailored analgesia in the peri-operative period. It provides support for the best anesthesia practices in an effort to avoid this complication which may have serious adverse effects for the patient.

The three essential components of conventional pressure monitoring systems are examined in Chapter 3, which can assist in the diagnosis of CS. In Chapter 4, the authors present their research on acute limb compartment syndrome (LCS), which when left untreated, can result in muscle necrosis and limb loss, and in severe cases, death. Both the prevention and treatment of compartment syndrome in severe cases is examined in detail. Chapter 5 focuses on lower limb compartment syndrome, a clinical entity resulting from increased pressure in a non-expansile tissue space, which is associated with significant morbidity and mortality. Chapter 6 focuses on Paraspinal Compartment Syndrome (PSCS), resulting in the "Bourdon tube effect." The last chapter, Chapter 8, reviews orbital compartment syndrome (OCS), a rare but treatable ophthalmic surgical emergency, caused most often by a retrobulbar hematoma, facial trauma being the most frequent etiological factor.

Chapter 1 - Acute compartment syndrome (ACS) was first described in 1875 by Dr. Richard Von Volkman. A vast body of research has been dedicated to ACS since that time and the syndrome's pathophysiology is almost uniformly agreed upon. For decades, intracompartmental pressure (ICP) monitoring has served as the gold-standard diagnostic modality for ACS. Despite its long-term use, several authors claim ICP monitoring lacks sensitivity and specificity resulting in both overdiagnosis and underdiagnosis - each with deleterious consequences. The targeted diagnosis and treatment of any disease must be cultivated from a comprehensive understanding of its pathophysiology. This chapter serves to review the current understanding of ACS's pathophysiology and highlight implications for the modernization of diagnosis and treatment.

Chapter 2 - Compartment Syndrome (CS) may develop following substantial injury to the muscles of the leg or arm. This injury may be related to recent surgery or may follow a crush or direct blunt trauma. Anesthesia may influence the development through the use of regional anesthesia, optimum blood pressure control and oxygen delivery, and tailored analgesia in the peri-operative period.

This chapter reviews the evidence relevant to how the anesthesiologist can influence the genesis of compartment syndrome. It provides support for best anesthesia practice in an effort to avoid this complication which may have serious adverse effects for the patient. The authors provide a structure which facilitates rapid and frequent evaluation of compartment pressures post-operatively, and discusses the management of CS after it has become established in the injured limb.

Chapter 3 - There are various underlying causes which initiate the sequence of events resulting in compartment syndrome including fractures, bleeding, tightly applied casts or extrinsic compression devices, burns and vigorous exercise. The common denominator appears to be an initial insult causing haemorrhage or oedema. This causes a rise in interstitial (tissue) fluid pressure in a closed osteofascial compartment (an anatomical space defined by rigid and unyielding boundaries). The result is vascular occlusion and subsequent reduced blood flow, the devastating sequelae of which are ischaemic necrosis of myoneural tissue and ultimate permanent contracture. This phenomenon was first described by Richard von Volkmann in 1881.

The degree of functional loss depends upon how quickly surgical decompression of the involved compartment is performed. Decompression itself can carry considerable morbidity with risks of infection and difficulty in wound closure requiring further plastic surgical procedures, thus prompt and accurate diagnosis is vital.

Early clinical findings of raised intracompartmental pressure include swelling, palpable tenseness over a muscle compartment and pain out of proportion to the injury or on passive stretch of the muscles in the compartment. Later signs include reduced or absent sensation, muscle paresis and loss of pulses. However these can often be subjective. For example, pain or nerve injury may be initiated by the initial direct trauma rather than compartment syndrome. Also, except in the case of major arterial injury, pulses may often be palpable even when a compartment syndrome is present. In particular, patient groups such as children, those with impaired or absent consciousness and in whom clinical findings are equivocal can be very difficult to diagnose on clinical grounds and therefore having an objective test to aid diagnosis and subsequent surgical management of acute compartment syndrome is imperative.

Chapter 4 - Acute limb compartment syndrome (LCS) is determined by edema and bleeding in a restrained muscle compartment limited by fascia and bone. LCS leads to muscle and nerve ischemia, threatening limb function and viability. The most frequent etiological factors are trauma and reperfusion, followed by acute arterial occlusion. Left untreated, LCS can result in muscle necrosis and limb loss and, in severe cases, renal impairment and even death. The mangled upper extremity is a limb with trauma involving bone, soft tissue, nerves and vessels. Arterial and venous injuries are present in 42% of patients with severe upper extremity trauma. Emergency reconstruction of the upper extremity after severe trauma has a better outcome than late reconstruction. Treatment includes tissue debridement, irrigation of traumatized tissue, stable fixation of bone, revascularization, nerve repair and coverage of soft tissue. The sequence of restoration of these anatomical structures depends on the ischemia time and the severity of injury. Preventing or treating compartment syndrome in severe cases is a cornerstone of the beginning of treatment. A gradual approach to the severe mangled extremity is further detailed.

Chapter 5 - Lower limb vascular injuries are often present in severe trauma. Frequently, the vascular lesions are associated with lower limb bone fractures, muscle contusion or rupture, burns and external limb compression. Among the most common causes are acute injuries by sharp objects, car accidents and fractures. Vein injuries are less often present but are possible in severe compartment syndrome. All these can lead to acute compartment syndrome due to intramuscular hematomas and soft tissue edema. Compartment syndrome of the lower limb is a clinical entity resulting from increased pressure in a non-expansile tissue space and is associated with significant morbidity and mortality. The diagnosis of compartment syndrome combined with vascular trauma in the lower limb is mostly clinical and by measurements of the compartment pressure. Diagnosis can be delayed in unconscious patients. It is of paramount importance to identify this problem and treat it as soon as possible. There are important predictor factors for fasciotomy: multi-system trauma, open fractures and knee dislocation associated with vascular injury. Herein we detail the step-by-step guide for identifying compartment syndrome in conscious and unconscious patients with lower limb vascular injuries and modalities of treatment.

Chapter 6 - Compartment Syndrome is a condition which signifies increased pressure in a confined anatomical space, resulting in compromised circulation and threatening the viability and function of the muscles. The paraspinal region is a potential area for developing compartment syndrome. The erector spinae muscles lay parallel to the dorsolumbar spine and have a curved tube shape, enclosed within a thin fascial layer. The increased intracompartmental pressures produce Paraspinal Compartment Syndrome (PSCS), resulting in the "Bourdon tube effect": the increased intratubal pressure straightens the curved tubes, producing rigidity of the paravertebral muscles and lordosis. Clinical signs include tenderness of the muscles and tenseness; severe pain during the muscle's contractions; and the appearance of pain during passive muscle stretch. Although usually this type of spinal compartment is acute and presents after surgery in this area, it can also become chronic. In chronic conditions, patients might present without any symptoms at rest, exercise-related back pain, a normal range of motion and no neurologic deficit in the lower limbs. This condition is less recognized in clinical practice.

Chapter 7 - Orbital compartment syndrome (OCS) is a rare but treatable ophthalmic surgical emergency, caused most often by a retrobulbar hematoma, facial trauma being the most frequent etiological factor. Iatrogenic causes are rarely discussed, and are most often overlooked. The prone position in long surgical procedures, such as posterior fossa or spinal surgery, has been recognized in the literature, but intracranial surgery for vascular or tumoral lesions along the sphenoid wing is rarely presented as an etiological factor for this frightening complication. Irreversible blindness can occur if the lateral canthotomy is not performed urgently. Multiple surgical procedures that can produce OCS are described in the literature. OCS can occur after endoscopic sinus surgery, transorbital neuroendoscopic surgery, cerebral aneurysm surgery, embolization of arterio-venous malformation or carotid-cavernous fistula, or any procedure performed in anterior skull base surgery.

It is for these reasons that we offer a comprehensive review of the orbital compartment syndrome from a neurosurgical point of view, focusing especially on neurosurgical procedures around the sphenoidal wing. We will not refer to lesions that secondarily involve the orbit, but will focus on those surgeries that address intracranial pathologies (vascular, tumoral or malformative), having OCS as a potential complication. Anatomical relationships, surgical procedures, possible pathophysiological mechanisms, clinical presentation and management of OCS are presented, based on actual literature and personal experience.

Recognition of OCS in the immediate postoperative period is of the outmost importance considering that, untreated, this complication may lead to visual loss. By being aware of the possible occurrence of OCS and by performing a relatively simple surgical procedure (canthotomy), blindness can be avoided.

In: Compartment Syndrome
Editor: Anna P. Henderson

ISBN: 978-1-63482-831-4

Chapter 1

The Pathophysiology of Acute Compartment Syndrome: Implications for Modern Diagnostics and Treatment

Alexander M. Crespo, Sanjit R. Konda and Kenneth A. Egol*
NYU Langone Medical Center, Hospital for Joint Diseases, NY, US

Abstract

Acute compartment syndrome (ACS) was first described in 1875 by Dr. Richard Von Volkman. A vast body of research has been dedicated to ACS since that time and the syndrome's pathophysiology is almost uniformly agreed upon. For decades, intracompartmental pressure (ICP) monitoring has served as the gold-standard diagnostic modality for ACS. Despite its long-term use, several authors claim ICP monitoring lacks sensitivity and specificity resulting in both overdiagnosis and underdiagnosis - each with deleterious consequences. The targeted diagnosis and treatment of any disease must be cultivated from a comprehensive understanding of its pathophysiology. This chapter serves to review the current understanding of ACS's pathophysiology and highlight implications for the modernization of diagnosis and treatment.

* Corresponding author: Kenneth.Egol@nyumc.org.

Introduction

Acute compartment syndrome (ACS) was first described 140 years ago by Dr. Richard Von Volkman in his work, "Non-Infective Ischemic Conditions of Various Fascial Compartments in the Extremities" [1]. Trauma, burns, reperfusion injury, drug overdose, prolonged surgery, and snake bites have been reported as causative events in acute compartment syndrome. Regardless of the cause, ACS develops when intracompartmental tissue swelling decreases the perfusion pressure, resulting in local ischemia and infarction.

The annual incidence for ACS is 7.3 per 100,000 males and 0.7 per 100,000 females [2]. There are over 200,000 cases of ACS diagnosed annually in the United States [3]. Males are considered more likely to develop the syndrome due to increased muscle bulk which decreases intracompartmental capacity. In addition to male gender, young patient age, long bone fracture, high energy mechanism, and major crushing injuries are all known risk factors for ACS. The mode of injury generally falls into one of three categories [2]:

1. Long bone fracture (70-75%)
2. Trauma without fracture (15-20%): direct or crushing blow, severe burns, vascular injury with intracompartmental bleeding
3. Non-traumatic: ischemia-reperfusion injury, bleeding disorders, nephrotic syndrome, IV drug use, prolonged limb compression, animal bites, etc.

If left untreated, ACS will result in muscle necrosis, contracture, and loss of function; some cases may require limb amputation. Prompt diagnosis and treatment is the only way to avoid such devastating sequelae.

Historically, the diagnosis of ACS has been primarily clinical and relies on the ability to obtain a history and physical exam. History and physical is aimed at identifying the "5 P's" of compartment syndrome: pain out of proportion to stimulus, pressure (palpable compartment tenseness), paresthesia, paralysis, and pulselessness. While these findings are often cited, their diagnostic sensitivity and specificity are quite poor [3-6]. Pain, often regarded as the paramount symptom in ACS, varies amongst patients and is difficult to objectively quantify. Furthermore, it is difficult to distinguish pain secondary to recent trauma from pain heralding the onset of an acute compartment syndrome. Finally, accurately assessing pain in the obtunded or comatose patient is nearly impossible. Palpable tenseness is a crude indicator of intracompartmental pressure and poorly evaluates deep tissue compartments. ACS may occur without ever causing pulselessness, paresthesias, or paralysis. When these findings do manifest, the surgeon should consider the following possibilities [3]:

1. There is a concomitant neurovascular injury requiring immediate attention
2. It is late in the disease process and chance of successful treatment is limited

Given the poor diagnostic accuracy and reproducibility of history and physical exam findings, physicians have made use of intracompartmental pressure (ICP) monitoring. This modality directly measures intracompartmental pressure and allows calculation of the perfusion pressure. Despite its current status as the diagnostic gold-standard for acute compartment syndrome, ICP monitoring has been reported to have poor diagnostic sensitivity and specificity [7-13].

Poor diagnostic ability coupled with devastating patient consequences in the case of a missed ACS fosters an environment where over diagnosis and overtreatment is common. ACS is a situation where diagnostic false-positives are tolerated but false-negatives are not, prompting physicians to "err on the side of caution" [6, 10]. The impetus for over diagnosis and treatment is strengthened by the fact that a missed ACS is the most common cause for a malpractice lawsuit against orthopaedic surgeons and often results in substantially higher indemnity payments [14, 15].

While "erring on the side of caution" is often necessary, it is certainly not benign. A diagnosis of ACS obliges treatment with fasciotomy. Although highly effective, fasciotomy is a morbid procedure requiring full release of skin, subcutaneous tissue, and fascia with delayed closure. As a result, patients are required to undergo a second operation to close the wound and are exposed to increased risk of infection while enduring longer and more expensive hospital stays [16, 17]. Ultimately, fasciotomy patients suffer from large scars and increased risk of permanent paresthesias, chronic venous insufficiency, tethered tendons, and chronic pain; these sequelae have been shown to cause patients to quit jobs and abandon hobbies [18].

Acute compartment syndrome creates a delicate scenario where the consequences of both under- and overdiagnosis are severe and unforgiving. Prompt, precise, and accurate diagnosis is the surgeon's only hope at successful navigation, yet few tools with these capabilities currently exist. Eliminating false-positive diagnoses or providing minimally invasive therapy early in the course of ACS promises to decrease the fasciotomy rate and increase quality of care. Novel diagnostic modalities with superior sensitivity and specificity may achieve this goal. The orthopaedic community has long been calling for such developments [4-6, 9, 10, 16, 17].

The Pathophysiology of Acute Compartment Syndrome

The pathophysiology of ACS is a vicious cycle of inflammation, edema, elevated ICP, decreased perfusion pressure, and low-flow ischemia incited by a sentinel event and ultimately resulting in tissue infarction (Figure 1).

Historically, the syndrome has been viewed as a "time-pressure" phenomenon whereby intracompartmental pressure is considered the paramount pathologic factor. According to Matsen, "Increased tissue pressure is, by definition, the central pathogenic factor in the compartmental syndrome" [19]. While increased ICP is certainly a requisite process in the pathology, it occurs early in the syndrome and does not obligatorily cause infarction of the intracompartmental contents. Ischemia, by definition, indicates a shortage of oxygen and glucose required for cellular viability and, if left untreated, will result in tissue infarction. As such, acute compartment syndrome should not be thought of as a "time-pressure" phenomenon but rather an ischemic phenomenon.

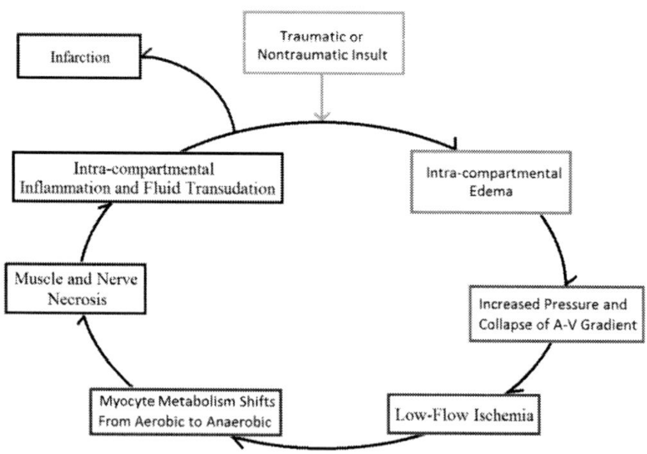

Figure 1. The vicious cycle of acute compartment syndrome.

I. The Inciting Event

As described earlier in this chapter, ACS may be caused by a variety of factors ranging from traumatic to atraumatic in nature. Though the causes are distinct in character, they each trigger a common pathophysiology unaltered by the inciting event.

II. Inflammation and Intracompartmental Edema

Trauma, reperfusion injury, or toxin exposure each result in local tissue damage and microvascular injury which serves to initiate and propagate the inflammatory response. The initial injury causes a cytokine release resulting in increased capillary permeability, fluid extravasation, recruitment of inflammatory cells, and further release of cytokines.

While ACS is an ischemic phenomenon, the role of inflammation should not be underestimated. Despite a dearth of research on acute compartment syndrome, the mechanism and impact of inflammation in ACS has only recently come to light as a result of several animal studies [20].

In an initial study to determine the role of inflammation, Lawendy et al., (unpublished data) induced compartment syndrome in neutropenic rats and normal rats. Intravital videomicroscopy (IVVM) was employed to visualize and quantify muscle injury and necrosis. The authors found that myocyte injury was reduced approximately 70% in neutropenic rats (lacking the ability to mount an inflammatory response). These findings suggested a previously underappreciated role of inflammation on cellular injury in ACS [20].

In a follow-up study, Lawendy et al., again utilized IVVM to visualize and study the microvascular response to acute compartment syndrome. The authors found that ACS results in a significant decrease in continuously perfused capillaries within the compartment, identifying the mechanism of low-flow ischemia. Perhaps more importantly, the authors also found that the mean number of adherent and activated leukocytes significantly increased in ACS while the number of rolling leukocytes did not. Leukocyte adherence and activation are caused by increased expression of integrins and immunoglobulins expressed by endothelial cells in a pro-inflammatory state. These observations characterize the early microvascular response to ACS: a decrease in capillary availability and an increase in leukocyte quantity and flow characteristics which are predicated on a pro-inflammatory environment [21].

The presence of a local and systemic pro-inflammatory state was investigated in a subsequent animal study (unpublished data) [20]. It was found that ACS resulted in a systemic increase of inflammatory cytokines such as IL-1β, GRO/KC, and TNF-α. Remote organ damage as a result of systemic inflammation was also measured in the liver, where necrotic hepatocytes were found after 2 hours of ACS. These findings suggest that ACS triggers not only a local inflammatory response, but a systemic response as well.

In a final study, indomethacin, a potent non-steroidal anti-inflammatory, was systemically delivered as a pre-treatment in an animal model of ACS and tissue injury was compared to a control group. Indomethacin inhibits cyclo-oxygenase thereby blocking the formation of cytotoxic enzymes and reactive oxygen species produced in the process of inflammation. The authors found that indomethacin treatment resulted in decreased apoptosis and cell damage while improving capillary perfusion [22].

Clinical data characterizing the inflammatory response to ACS are limited by the acute nature of the disease. Nonetheless, these recent in vivo animal studies have begun to highlight the previously underappreciated role of inflammation in ACS. Continued research aimed at modulating inflammation may yield promising non-invasive medical treatment of the syndrome.

III. Increased Intracompartmental Pressure and Collapse of the Arteriovenous Gradient

Perfusion is defined as the process of delivering arterial blood to a capillary bed, allowing for diffusion of oxygen and nutrients. Perfusion requires a pressure gradient between the high-pressure arterial system and low-pressure venous system. This allows delivery of oxygenated blood to a capillary bed and removal of deoxygenated blood.

The inflammatory process elucidated earlier causes increased capillary permeability and fluid extravasation within a compartment. The resulting interstitial edema and cellular swelling increases the volume of intracompartmental contents. As the volume approaches the capacity of an unyielding fascial compartment, the intracompartmental pressure obligatorily rises.

The arteriovenous pressure gradient theory of ACS was introduced by Matsen and Krugmire in 1978 [23]. It is based on the premise that increased intracompartmental pressure is transmitted across thin-walled intracompartmental venules thereby raising intraluminal venous pressures.

Increasing venous pressure results in further fluid accumulation via hydrostatic transudate as well as a diminished pressure gradient between arterial and venous systems. The loss of an aterio-venous pressure gradient impedes perfusion and results in local ischemia. The IVVM studies mentioned earlier, in which ACS significantly decreased continuously perfused capillaries, and several other studies give credence to this theory [21, 24].

Acceptance of this theory led to a change in how ACS is diagnosed using ICP monitoring. Originally, absolute ICP > 40mmHg was the threshold for diagnosis. As the arteriovenous gradient theory gained traction, authors began advocating use of the "differential pressure" or "delta pressure", defined as the difference between diastolic blood pressure (DBP) and ICP ($\Delta P = DBP - ICP$). Popularized by Whitesides et al., this measurement acknowledges the importance of perfusion in ACS and attempts to identify collapse of the arteriovenous gradient [25]. Today, this is the commonly used measurement in diagnosing ACS.

IV. Low-Flow Ischemia

Ischemia is the central pathologic factor in acute compartment syndrome. Collapse of the arteriovenous gradient creates an environment where perfusion is diminished, but not completely inhibited; a process termed "low-flow" ischemia. Intracompartmental pressures rarely exceed that of systolic blood pressure, meaning that blood flow into the compartment is not completely blocked.

Low-flow ischemia differs from absolute ischemia (arterial occlusion) in subtle but important ways. Most importantly, there is still arterial flow into the compartment. This is why pulselessness (despite being one of the "5 P's" of diagnosing ACS) is almost never encountered in ACS; in fact a finding of non-palpable pulses should prompt consideration of an arterial injury rather than ACS. Furthermore, low-flow ischemia means that oxygen and glucose are still supplied to the tissue, albeit at levels non-conducive to myocyte viability over a prolonged period of time. Finally, it is possible that systemic intravenous therapies may still enter the compartment since blood flow is not completely occluded. Nonetheless, "low-flow" arterial influx is still unable to meet the metabolic demands of muscle, thus causing ischemia. The lack of glucose and oxygen forces myocytes to transition from aerobic to anaerobic metabolism in order to survive in an ischemic environment.

V. Myocyte Transition from Aerobic to Anaerobic Metabolism

In the time between onset of low-flow ischemia and infarction, myocytes undergo a predictable change in metabolic processes to survive in an ischemic environment. At low oxygen saturation the ability of mitochondrial enzymes to reduce O2 to H2O becomes substrate limited by O2 availability, resulting in the need for supplemental glycolysis to support ATP production [26]. As glycolysis persists at an increased rate, the cell's supply of NAD+ must be regenerated by conversion of pyruvate to lactic acid. As a result, myocyte viability is largely dependent on access to glucose and ability to maintain glycolysis [26]. Prolonged low-flow ischemia impedes ability to maintain glycolysis, resulting in diminished ATP availability and ultimately, infarction.

Lindsay et al., studied the effect of prolonged ischemia and its impact on muscle metabolism. They found that ischemia results in complete depletion of creatine phosphate and adenosine triphosphate (ATP). This resulted in 51% muscle necrosis at 5 hour [27]. A separate study noted similar findings and determined that ATP levels were reduced by 80% after 6 hours of ischemia [28]. Both authors concluded that myocytes are only able to withstand anaerobic metabolism for a finite period of time, and length of the ischemic period may be the ultimate predictor of infarction.

A pilot study by our group has demonstrated ischemia-induced changes in metabolite kinetics (glucose and lactate) measured by microdialysis in ACS [29]. In a rabbit model, interstitial lactate underwent a steady increase throughout the trial with a significant ischemic response between 4-6 hours (969% increase from baseline) (Figures 2&3).

Although interstitial lactate rose dramatically throughout the trial, indicating the presence of anaerobic metabolism, it should be noted that glucose levels never reached "0". This is likely due to the presence of "low-flow" ischemia and not complete arterial occlusion. If "no-flow" ischemia had taken place, a complete utilization of glucose would be expected and there would be undetectable levels of the substrate.

These aforementioned studies demonstrate a clear transition from aerobic to anaerobic metabolism caused by ACS. Anaerobic metabolism can only sustain myocyte viability for a finite period of time before energy demands are no longer met and cell death occurs. Inability to release intracompartmental pressure and eliminate low-flow ischemia in a timely fashion inevitably leads to the final step of ACS: infarction.

VI. Infarction of Intracompartmental Contents

The natural history of acute compartment syndrome yields infarction of the intracompartmental contents eventually followed by fibrosis and contracture. While ischemia is reversible with little consequence, infarction is irreversible and will result in functional loss. In essence, the pathophysiology is similar to a myocardial infarction where prolonged ischemia results in cell death. The time between ischemic onset and myocyte necrosis is a "golden window" where time to intervention is critical [3, 4, 6]; much like myocardial infarction, "time equals muscle".

Clinical and basic science research demonstrates that striated muscle cells can tolerate warm ischemia for three to eight hours before infarction [30]. Clinically, intervention within 6 hours of ischemic onset is the goal. There are a myriad of factors that affect myocyte tolerability of ischemia which include: extent of initial injury, presence of concomitant injuries, hemodynamic status of the patient, proportion of red-muscle fibers within the muscle belly, etc. Furthermore, much of the basic science research in this realm has been extrapolated from tourniquet models and not ACS based models. Although there are similarities between the two models, there are also important pathophysiologic differences. Heppenstall et al., demonstrated that increased ICP causes a metabolic insult that acts synergistically with ischemia to produce more profound cellular deterioration than ischemia alone (tourniquet models) [31-33]. As such, ACS may shorten the "golden window". A large retrospective review by Vaillancourt et al., showed that ACS-induced necrosis can occur rapidly and was evident in some patients at 3 hours from the time of injury [34]. Ultimately, early diagnosis and treatment is essential to procuring a positive outcome.

Histologically, striated muscle infarction follows the common phases of wound healing seen in other tissues: inflammation, proliferation, and maturation. The inflammatory phase occurs on the order of hours to days. Initially, myocytes undergo intracellular movement of sacrolemmal nuclei, glycogen depletion, increased calcium content, atrophy, and apoptosis. The interstitium is then infiltrated with acute inflammatory cells in which neutrophils and macrophages are the predominant cells at work and serve to autolyse any necrotic tissue. The proliferative phase occurs between 7-30 days and is characterized by fibroblasts actively forming granulation tissue, which is mainly comprised of collagen. Myocytes, like neurons, have poor ability to regenerate and proliferate. Therefore, the proliferative phase is heavily dominated by fibrosis while myocyte regeneration is minimal; this makes full return of function nearly impossible. Maturation occurs over several months and consists of collagen remodeling and contraction. The end result is a scarred and contracted muscle belly dominated by fibrosis and rendered functionally useless [35-37].

Intracompartmental Pressure Monitoring

The clinical diagnosis of ACS, using the "5 P's" mentioned earlier, has been shown to be a poor indicator of the syndrome [5, 38]. This has led to the adoption of intracompartmental pressure monitoring as an adjunct to the clinical exam. ICP monitoring is predicated on the acknowledgement that ACS is a "pressure phenomena" and provides an objective method of evaluating patients at risk. This technique and the ICP threshold for diagnosing ACS have evolved substantially over the past 40 years.

Direct compartment measurement using a wick-catheter was first popularized by Mubarak and Owen in the late 1970's [39-41]. The wick catheter is comprised of strands of wet fibers connected proximally to a pressure transducer. The distal end is implanted into the tissue of interest. The wet fibers establish a continuous fluid column between the compartment and pressure transducer so that pressure is transmitted across the catheter and analyzed by the transducer. The side portal needle system (Stryker® needle) is based on this concept and is currently the most commonly used tool to measure ICP.

In the original clinical study using a wick-catheter, Mubarak et al., used an ICP threshold of greater than 30 mmHg as an indication for fasciotomy. In unaffected patients, the normal compartment pressure was 0-10 mmHg. In sixteen patients clinically suspected of having an acute compartment syndrome, but with ICP pressures less than 30 mmHg, fasciotomy was withheld and none developed sequelae of ACS. Furthermore, intra-operative wick-catheter monitoring showed a decrease in ICP after fasciotomy and was used to ensure adequate decompression [40].

Eventually, it became apparent that a patient's ability to tolerate elevated ICP is markedly variable and the "30 mmHg" cutoff did not universally indicate an acute compartment syndrome. Shortly after the publication of Mubarak's work, Matsen et al., demonstrated that muscle and nerve integrity is maintained at higher ICP elevations. They suggested an absolute pressure of 45 mmHg was a more appropriate threshold for diagnosing ACS [42].

While Mubarak and Matsen were investigating the utility of absolute ICP measurement, another theory was emerging. Whitesides et al., considered the role of the patient's hemodynamic status in tolerating increased ICP. In accordance with the arteriovenous gradient theory, the group hypothesized that ischemia commences when compartmental perfusion is limited. Perfusion is measured by calculating the "perfusion pressure" (also referred to as "differential pressure" or "ΔP") which is the difference between diastolic blood pressure and absolute ICP (ΔP = DBP – ICP). Whitesides et al., stated that ischemia begins when ΔP is between 10-30 mmHg [25], and this report led to adoption of "differential pressure" monitoring for diagnosing ACS.

Like absolute pressure monitoring, differential pressure monitoring has failed to yield a decisive threshold for diagnosis. A histologic study by Heckman et al., showed no muscle damage with ΔP > 20 mmHg, minimal damage when ΔP was between 20 and 10 mmHg, scattered areas of infarction when ΔP was between 10 and 0 mmHg, and widespread infarction when ΔP = 0 mmHg. They recommended a diagnostic criteria of ΔP = 10-20 mmHg [36]. A subsequent clinical study by McQueen et al., found that using a threshold of ΔP < 30 mmHg led to no missed cases of ACS and recommended that decompression be performed if the differential pressure drops below this point [44]. Currently, there are multiple ICP definitions used as an indication for fasciotomy (Table 1). Lack of a universal ICP threshold for diagnosing ACS makes ICP monitoring a confusing and "controversial component" in evaluating at-risk patients [6]; one study has shown that 42% of surgeons are unsure what ICP level requires fasciotomy [45].

The use of ICP monitoring as a diagnostic tool is further complicated by variations in technique and patient characteristics. ICP measurements have been shown to vary within an injured compartment. Measurements have been shown to be significantly different - as much as 20 mmHg - when the probe is placed within an area just 5cm from the fracture site [43]. Even small changes in position of the leg (dorsiflexion/plantarflexion of the ankle and flexion/extension of the knee) have been shown to significantly alter ICP [46]. Patients with antecedent ischemia (peripheral vascular disease) are significantly more sensitive to increases in ICP than those with normal vasculature [47]. Simple elevation of the extremity can reduce tolerability of muscle for increased ICP [48]. Finally, analgesics and epidurals used for post-traumatic pain control are known to increase local blood flow secondary to sympathetic blockade and can lead to variance in tolerability of increased IC [6,49]. These relatively minute differences amongst patients, coupled with a lack of uniform ICP threshold, have caused many to question the diagnostic utility of ICP monitoring.

Although ICP measurement is the most widely studied and commonly used technique for diagnosing ACS, it has been heavily criticized for having poor diagnostic sensitivity and specificity in the past decade [7-13]. The estimated specificity of the "ΔP < 30mmHg" threshold is less than 65% [10]. One study followed ICP measurements on a cohort of patients with tibial shaft fracture and not suspected to have ACS and found that 84% of the patients had at least one measurement that would have indicated them for fasciotomy [12]. This trend was confirmed in the only randomized control trial comparing ICP monitoring to clinical evaluation alone; the authors found that ICP monitoring would have resulted in 18% of patients receiving an unnecessary fasciotomy [11]. The low reliability of pressure monitoring has resulted in inconsistent quality of care. A study of surgeon behavior at a single institution revealed surgeon fasciotomy rates range from 2-24% yet the low fasciotomy surgeons did suffer from missed diagnoses. The results suggest that surgeon reliance on a test prone to false positives significantly increases the fasciotomy rate [50]. Only one retrospective study exists demonstrating the effective diagnostic utility of ICP monitoring; the authors showed a specificity of 93%, sensitivity of 98%, positive predictive value of 93% and negative predictive value of 99% [51].

Despite its flaws, ICP monitoring is the most readily available and studied method currently available to diagnose ACS. Since no specific, reliable, and reproducible test exists, the surgeon is placed in a difficult position when evaluating patients at risk for ACS. The finding of elevated ICP pressure effectively obligates fasciotomy, regardless of overall clinical suspicion. Opting to forego compartment pressure evaluation exposes the patient to risk of negative sequelae. Underdiagnosis and overdiagnosis are equally maleficent. As such, the diagnostic process must have excellent accuracy and reliability. The true breakthrough in early and accurate diagnosis of ACS will likely come from novel modalities capable of determining the degree of ischemia within a compartment rather than its abnormal pressure state [4,9].

Table 1. Indications for fasciotomy

Absolute ICP Measurement	Differential Pressure Measurement
ICP > 30 mmHg(Mubarak et al.)	ΔP = 10-20 mmHg(Heckman et al.)
ICP > 45 mmHg(Matsen et al.)	ΔP < 30 mmHg(McQueen et al.)

On the Horizon: New Diagnostic Modalities

The limitations of ICP monitoring have spurred investigations into new diagnostic techniques in ACS over the past decade. Newer modalities, such as near-infrared spectroscopy, microdialysis, and ultrafiltration each aim to improve diagnostic accuracy and reliability. Despite their relative infancy, each modality has potential to improve quality of care in acute compartment syndrome.

Near-Infrared Spectroscopy (NIRS)

Near-infrared spectroscopy is a method using the near-infrared region of the electromagnetic spectrum (800nm – 2500nm) to evaluate energy states of a given molecule. The technology has broad applications ranging from astronomy to medicine. In medicine, NIRS's primary application is based on the fact that distinct biologic molecules change their optical properties when bound to oxygen. This change is readily apparent when observing the color difference between crimson hued deoxygenated (venous) blood and bright red oxygenated (arterial) blood [52]. The optical change occurs because deoxyhemoglobin and oxyhemoglobin differ in optical absorbance patterns, causing color change. Spectroscopy is capable of quantifying these optic differences and directly evaluating the oxygenation (stO2) of a given tissue.

NIRS relies on Beer's law, which dictates that light transmission through a mixed solution decreases as the concentration of a solute increases. Since deoxyhemoglobin and oxyhemoglobin have different absorbance patterns, their relative concentrations can be determined by spectroscopy [52]. Clinically, the device functions as follows: a source generating NIR light of a given wavelengths is placed on the skin overlying the tissue of interest and secured with a sticker to block ambient light. On its way through tissue, NIR interacts with multiple chromophores, of which hemoglobin is most important. NIR light is then reflected back to the skin probe which quantifies the spectral differences between oxyhemoglobin and deoxyhemoglobin, providing direct insight to the tissue's oxygenation status. Originally, these properties made NIRS popular in the neurosurgical setting as a method of evaluating trans-cranial cerebral oxygenation [53-55].

NIRS was first investigated as a tool for diagnosing ACS in 1999 when Garr et al., hypothesized that measuring oxygen concentration in venous blood provides insight to a tissue's oxygen extraction. In an animal model, the authors placed NIRS probes over the anterior compartment and created a model of ACS. They found a significant inverse correlation between absolute ICP and oxygenation. Likewise, there was a significant correlation between ΔP and oxygenation. Lastly, tissue oxygenation was a better predictor of neuromuscular impairment than perfusion pressure [52]. A follow-up animal study confirmed the responsiveness of NIRS in the setting of hypotension and hypoxemia [56]. Finally, in a simulated model involving human volunteers, NIRS was shown to be more sensitive in detecting lower leg ischemia than ICP monitoring [57].

In 2000, the first clinical study of NIRS's ability to detect ischemic changes in ACS was performed. NIRS probes were used to measure pre and post-surgical oxygenation in 9 patients with confirmed ACS based on clinical and ICP evaluation. Oxygenation in the affected limb was a mean 56 +/- 27% at diagnosis and improved to 82 +/- 16% after fasciotomy [58]. A follow-up clinical study confirmed the responsiveness of NIRS by showing that oxygenation decreased by 10-16% in limbs with ACS when compared to the unaffected contralateral limb [59].

While the results of Shuler and Giannotti's studied were promising, some concern over the utility of NIRS has arisen. A recent study by Bariteau et al., has demonstrated no reliable correlation between NIRS evaluation and ICP pressure findings. The authors found that several patients had clinical and ICP findings indicative of an acute compartment syndrome, yet did not demonstrate decreased oxygenation via NIRS evaluation. This inconsistency led to premature closure of the study [60].

NIRS evaluation is complicated by two separate influences: the pathophysiology of acute trauma and mechanical limitations of the technology itself. Acute trauma has been shown to cause a local hyperemic response at the injured area, which is detectable by NIRS [61]. A local hyperemic response may cause an apparent raise in stO2, as detected by NIRS, despite concurrent elevated ICP; this may cause the surgeon to errantly exclude a diagnosis of ACS. NIRS has also been shown to have a tissue penetration of only 3cm, making evaluation of deep tissue compartments (the deep posterior compartment of the leg) difficult. Furthermore, NIRS data may be altered by the presence of other chromophores (melanin) and hematoma formation. This may lead to variation in normal stO2 readings amongst patients of darker skin tone and those with extensive injury [60,61].

Research regarding the diagnostic ability of NIRS in ACS is still ongoing. There is hope that continuous NIRS monitoring, as opposed to isolated measurements performed in prior studies, may avoid difficulties interpreting data in light of the hyperemic response [61]. Despite its limitations, NIRS represents a shift in diagnosing ACS as it evaluates the presence of ischemia rather than isolated elevation of ICP. Further research will continue to determine the value of this noninvasive modality in diagnosing ACS.

Microdialysis

Microdialysis is a technique consisting of a probe with a semi-permeable membrane designed to function as a capillary [62]. The membrane is perfused with a fluid isotonic to the interstitium allowing for diffusion of molecules across the membrane, down the concentration gradient. This technique allows for frequent monitoring of chemical changes in the interstitium, which reflect intracellular changes [63]. Furthermore, the perfusate may be instilled with high-concentration therapeutic agents that diffuse into the interstitial environment. This unique property allows microdialysis to be both diagnostic and therapeutic.

Like NIRS, microdialysis has clinical origins in the neurosurgical setting where it was used to detect cerebral ischemia after a stroke. In more recent years, microdialysis has also been used experimentally to investigate muscle tissue metabolism in a variety of ischemic settings. Pojar et al., used this technique to monitor peripheral tissue metabolism in off-pump vs. on-pump coronary bypass surgery [64]. Korth et al., have used microdialysis to analyze metabolism changes in skeletal muscle caused by use of a tourniquet in orthopaedic surgeries [65]. Muller et al., have also utilized microdialysis to monitor metabolite kinetics in skeletal muscle during ischemia and reperfusion [66]. In each of the aforementioned studies, microdialysis detected similar decreases in interstitial glucose concentration and increases in lactate following the onset of ischemia. Furthermore, several studies have shown that concentration changes of lactate and glucose during ischemia correlate with the severity of ischemic tissue damage [66]. The ability to detect metabolic changes indicative of local ischemia makes microdialysis a promising tool in the diagnosis of ACS.

A pilot study by our group has demonstrated that by monitoring skeletal muscle interstitial glucose and lactate kinetics, microdialysis is capable of detecting ischemic change in ACS [29]. We found that interstitial lactate underwent a steady increase throughout the trial with a significant ischemic response between 4-6 hours (969% increase from baseline) (Figures 2&3). These results are consistent with prior studies demonstrating myocyte viability dramatically decreases after 6 hours of ischemia [27, 28].

Our data also revealed that mean intra-compartmental glucose undergoes an initial surge before gradually returning to baseline. The lactate-glucose ratio was 1.4 at baseline and peaked at 15.9, indicating that anaerobic metabolism is outpacing glucose supply. There was a high correlation (r=0.91) between percent change in local glucose and lactate levels (from immediately previous values) in the first 60 minutes. The correlation gradually diminished after 2 hours (r=0.65) and remained steady over the remainder of the trial (r=0.65 at 8 hours) (Figure 3).

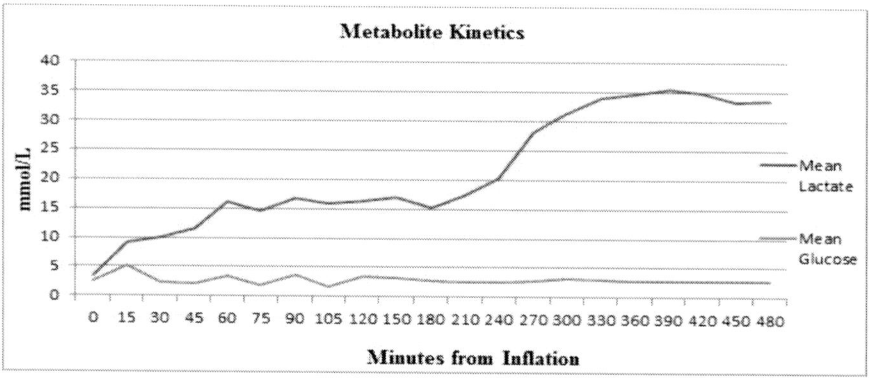

Figure 2. Interstitial Metabolite Kinetics.

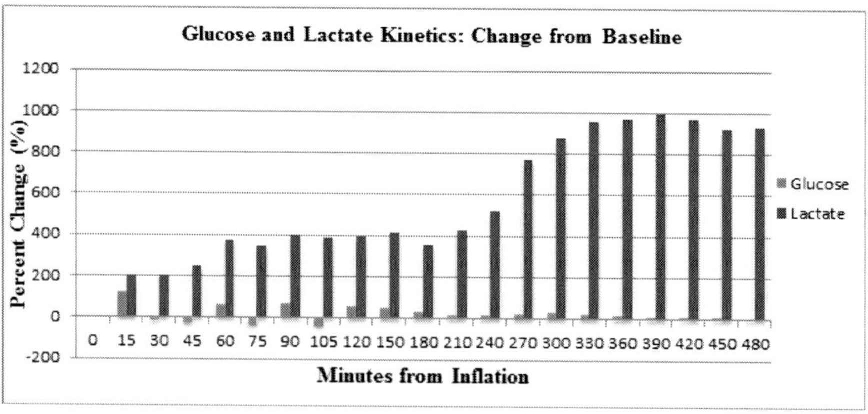

Figure 3. Glucose and Lactate Percent Change from Baseline.

This work represents the first report of both glucose and lactate kinetics in the setting of ACS. Our results support and expand upon prior work demonstrating that local glucose and pH monitoring using implantable probes may identify early onset ischemia [67,68]. Although not new to clinical use, using microdialysis to diagnose acute compartment syndrome is in its infancy. The technology has a proven ability to detect local ischemic change in a variety of tissues and offers a promising application to acute compartment syndrome. Microdialysis's ability to provide immediate and continuous data, coupled with the capability to locally delivery therapy, further bolsters its promise. Nonetheless, an abundance of clinical work is needed.

Tissue Ultrafiltration

Tissue ultrafiltration (TUF) is a technology in which small hollow fibers are implanted into tissue for the removal of interstitial fluid. The fibers are connected to a negative pressure device allowing suction-based removal of the fluid. Historically, TUF has been used experimentally to reduce tissue edema in skin flaps and cerebral models [69-71]. Recent research has been dedicated to exploring TUF's role as a diagnostic and therapeutic modality.

TUF was first investigated in a porcine model of acute compartment syndrome. A crush injury was induced bilaterally with unilateral TUF treatment to allow internal experimental control. TUF removed a mean 0.9 mL of fluid from the compartment and reduced ICP by an average of 10 mmHg when compared to the non-treatment side. This resulted in improved perfusion pressure and limited myocyte damage. Fluid analysis revealed substantial increases in lactate dehydrogenase (LDH) and creatine phosphokinase (CPK) [37].

A follow-up clinical study yielded similar results. A total of 10 patients with tibial shaft fractures were included in the study. TUF removed a mean of 1.9 mL of fluid which was associated with decreases in ICP, improvement in perfusion pressure, and decrease in LDH and CPK [72]. Although early results of TUF have been promising, further investigations are needed. A randomized control trial comparing TUF to isolated ICP monitoring is underway [72].

While TUF has been shown to provide insight to local tissue changes in acute compartment syndrome, the ultimate goal of this research is to demonstrate its utility as a therapeutic modality. ACS is known to result in both interstitial fluid accumulation as well as intracellular swelling. ICP elevation is thought to be more dependent on tissue swelling than interstitial fluid accumulation. As such, TUF's ability to significantly alter ICP may be limited. While TUF treatment has been associated with decreased ICP, there is no evidence suggesting that treatment results in a more rapid ICP reduction than the natural history of ACS alone. Results from randomized clinical trials with adequate power are needed before definitive conclusions can be made.

Summary

The ideal diagnostic modality for acute compartment syndrome will evaluate ischemic change, demonstrate superior accuracy and reproducibility, allow for continuous monitoring, provide immediate bedside feedback, be minimally invasive, and provide a therapeutic function (Figure 4).

Near-infrared spectroscopy, microdialysis, and tissue ultrafiltration each has the potential to alter the way ACS is diagnosed and treated. By definition, ACS is a result of elevated intracompartmental pressure. However, it is evident that measuring ICP alone suffers from poor sensitivity and specificity. By measuring local oxygenation (NIRS), metabolite kinetics (microdialysis), or release of intracellular contents (TUF), these modalities represent a promising paradigm shift: they acknowledge that ischemia is the paramount pathologic factor at work in ACS. By moving away from ICP measurement and towards identifying ischemic onset, these novel modalities represent a promising future in the early diagnosis and management of acute compartment syndrome.

	Evaluates Ischemia	Accurate and Reproducible	Continuous Monitoring	Bedside Feedback	Non-invasive	Potentially Therapeutic
Intra-compartmental Pressure Monitoring	✗	✗	✓	✓	✗	✗
Microdialysis	✓	?	✓	✓	✗	✓
Near-Infrared Spectroscopy (NIRS)	✓	?	✓	✓	✓	✗
Tissue Ultrafiltration	✓	?	✗	✗	✗	✓

Figure 4. A summation of diagnostic techniques for acute compartment syndrome.

The Future of Treatment

Fasciotomy is a surgical procedure requiring full release of the skin, subcutaneous tissue, and fascia. Urgent fasciotomy for the treatment of patients with ACS is required to alleviate ICP and prevent tissue infarction. Despite being the only accepted treatment for ACS, fasciotomy is highly invasive and associated with substantial morbidity, increased length of stay, and significant cost of treatment [16-18]. Advances in treatment which serve to decrease the fasciotomy rate while preserving tissue viability and function may further improve quality of care.

Modulating ACS Pathophysiology

Treatment via fasciotomy stems from the dogma that "increased intracompartmental pressure = acute compartment syndrome". However, as shown in Figure 1, increased intracompartmental pressure is only one step in the multifaceted evolution of ACS. Each step along the "vicious cycle" of ACS represents a potential therapeutic target for disease modulation. The ultimate question is, "How does one break the pathophysiologic cycle of ACS?"

The contribution of acute inflammation to the pathophysiology of ACS has been extensively investigated in recent years. Ongoing research has identified the primary role leukocytes play in inciting microvascular dysfunction as well as exacerbating tissue injury in ACS [73]. While still in early stages, this research may ultimately identify disease modulating therapies that subvert the need for surgical intervention.

Limiting inflammation based injury is contingent upon either halting the infiltration of inflammatory cells or limiting their cytotoxic effect. An increase in local activated leukocytes has been associated with increased muscle damage [21]. Manjoo et al., investigated the therapeutic potential of the non-steroidal anti-inflammatory, indomethacin. The group found that pretreating animals with indomethacin before raising ICP reduced white cell activation and preserved muscle. Indomethacin is thought to have a two-pronged protective effect: it limits white cell infiltration as well as limits the production of cytotoxic reactive oxygen species (ROS). The net effect is a reduction in myocyte apoptosis and preservation of muscle function [22]. Similar work with N-acetylcystiene (NAC), an antioxidant commonly used to combat hepatocyte injury in acetaminophen overdose, has also been performed. NAC was found to reduce neutrophil respiratory burst, and thus the creation of ROS, as well as preserve myocyte contractility [74].

Modulating microvascular dysfunction may also offer protective effects against ACS. Carbon monoxide (CO) inhalation therapy has been shown to alleviate microvascular dysfunction caused by systemic and local inflammation secondary to ischemia-reperfusion injury [75-77]. This finding lead to the development of CO-releasing molecules (CO-RM's), which deliver CO in a controlled and targeted manner [78,79]. CO-RM's were used in an animal model of ACS and found to result in improved capillary perfusion, diminished parenchymal injury, decreased leukocyte adherence, and decreased markers of inflammation [73].

While the body of research regarding disease modification of ACS is limited, it demonstrates an alternative approach to treatment. Developing a neoadjuvant therapy administered early in the evolution of ACS, when the diagnosis remains unclear, could ultimately lower the fasciotomy rate. Nonetheless, the clinical utility of indomethacin, N-acetylcysteine, and CO-RMs remains to be proven.

Conclusion

Acute compartment syndrome is a well known entity with a long history of controversy regarding diagnostic accuracy. Over a century's worth of work has been dedicated to understanding and treating this condition, and yet we are left with relatively limited and simplistic methods of diagnosis and treatment. Like any disease, progress in diagnosis and treatment is predicated on intimate understanding of the underlying pathophysiology. The future of diagnostic accuracy and subsequent treatment of acute compartment syndrome with several promising diagnostic and therapeutic modalities is promising.

References

[1] von Volkmann; R. Veilletzungen und Krankenheiten der Berwegungsorgane. In: von Pithe F, Billroth T. Stuttgart, Verlag von Ferdinand Enke, eds. Handbuch der Allgemeinen und Speziellen Chirurgs. Zweiter Band, Zweiter Abteilung, Abschmitt V, Ersted haft: 188, 234-920.

[2] McQueen, MM; Gaston, P; Court-Brown, CM. Acute compartment syndrome: who is at risk? *J Bone Joint Surg Br.*, 2000, 82(2), 200-3.

[3] Konstantakos, EK; Dalstrom, DJ; Nelles, ME; et al. Diagnosis and management of extremity compartment syndromes: an orthopaedic perspective. *Amer Surg.*, 2007, 73(12), 1199-1209.

[4] Elliott, KB; Johnstone, AJ. Diagnosing Acute Compartment Syndrome. *J Bone Joint Surg Br.*, 2003, 85B, 625-32.

[5] Ulmer, T. The clinical diagnosis of acute compartment syndrome of the lower leg: are clinical findings predictive of the disorder? *J Orthop Trauma.*, 2002, 16(8), 572-7.

[6] Taylor, RM; Sullivan, MP; Mehta, S. Acute compartment syndrome: obtaining diagnosis, providing treatment, and minimizing medicolegal risk. *Curr Rev Musculoskelet Med.*, 2012, 5, 206-13.

[7] Van Zyl, AA; Van den berg, JL. Is compartment pressure measurement really necessary? *J Bone Joint Surg Br.*, 1989, (71), 713.

[8] Triffit, PD; Konig, WM; Harper, MR; et al. Compartment pressures after closed tibial shaft fracture. Their relation to functional outcome. *J Bone Joint Surg Br.*, 1992, 76, 1285-92.

[9] Janzing, HM; Broos, PL. Routine monitoring of compartment pressure in patients with tibial fractures: beware of overtreatment! *Injury*. 2001, 32, 415-21.

[10] Nelson, JA. Compartment pressure measurements have poor specificity for compartment syndrome in the traumatized limb. *J Emerg Med*. 2013, 44(5), 1039-44.

[11] Harris, IA; Kadir, A; Donald, G. Continuous compartment pressure monitoring for tibia fractures: does it influence outcome? *J Trauma*. 2006, 60, 1330-35.

[12] Prayson, MJ; Chen, JL; Hampers, D; et al. Baseline compartment pressure measurements in isolated lower extremity fractures without clinical compartment syndrome. *J Trauma.*, 2006, 60, 1037-40.

[13] White, TO; Howell, GED; Will, EM; et al. Elevated intramuscular pressures do not influence outcome after tibial fracture. *J Trauma*. 2003, 55, 1133–1138.

[14] Templeman, DVT; Schmidt, R. Economic Costs of Missed Compartment Syndromes. *Annual Meeting of American Academy of Orthopaedic Surgeons*. San Francisco, California. 1993.

[15] Bhattacharyya, T; Vrahas, MS. The medical-legal aspects of compartment syndrome. *J Bone Joint Surg Am.*, 2004, 86A:864-8.

[16] Crespo, AM; Manoli, A; Konda, SR; Egol, KA. Development of compartment syndrome negatively impacts length of stay and cost following tibia fracture. *J Orthop Trauma.*, 2014, Epub ahead of print.

[17] Schmidt, AH. The impact of compartment syndrome on hospital length of stay and charges among adult patients admitted with fracture of the tibia. *J Orthop Trauma.*, 2011, 25(6), 355-7.

[18] Fitzgerald, AM; Gatson, P; Wilson, Y; et al. Long-term sequelae of fasciotomy wounds. *Br J Plast Surg.*, 2000, 53(8), 690-3.

[19] Matsen, FA. Compartmental syndrome. A unified concept. *Clin Orthop Relat Res.*, 1975, (113), 8-14.

[20] Harvey, EJ; Sanders, DW; Shuler, MS; et al. What's new in acute compartment syndrome? *J Orthop Trauma.*, 2012, 26(12), 699-702.

[21] Lawendy, AR; Sanders, DW; Bihari, A; et al. Compartment syndrome-induced microvascular dysfunction: an experimental model. *Can J Surg.*, 2011, 54(3), 194-200.

[22] Manjoo, A; Sanders, D; Lawendy, A; et al. Indomethacin reduces cell damage: shedding new light on compartment syndrome. *J Orthop Trauma*. 2010, 24, 526–529.

[23] Matsen, FA III; Krugmire, RB. Compartmental syndromes. *Surg Gynecol Obstet*, 1978, 147, 943-9.

[24] Vollmar, B; Westermann, S; Menger, MD. Microvascular response to compartment syndrome-like external pressure elevation: an in vivo fluorescence microscopic study in the hamster striated muscle. *J Trauma.*, 1999, 46(1), 91-6.

[25] Whitesides, TE; Haney, TC; Morimoto, K; Harada, H. Tissue pressure measurements as a determinant for the need for fasciotomy. *Clin Orthop.* 1975, 113, 43-51.

[26] Clanton, TL; Klawitter, PF. Invited review: Adaptive responses of skeletal muscle to intermittent hypoxia: the known and the unknown. *J Appl Physiol*, 2001. 90(6), p. 2476-87.

[27] Lindsay, T; Liauw, F; Romaschin, S; et al. The effect of ischemia/reperfusion of adenine nucleotide metabolism and xanthine oxidase production in skeletal muscle. *J Vasc Surg*, 1990. 12, p. 8-15.

[28] Hayes, G; Liauw, S; Romaschin, A; et al. Separation of reperfusion injury from ischemia-induced necrosis. *Surg Forum*, 1988. 39, p. 306-8.3

[29] Crespo, AM; Konda, SR; Goch, AM; Egol, KA. Microdialysis detects ischemic change early in acute compartment syndrome: an improvement over standard intra-compartmental pressure monitoring. Sir Robert Jones

Annual Research Symposium. NYU Langone Medical Center, Hospital for Joint Diseases. May 2015.

[30] Hargens, AR; Schmidt, DA; Evans, KL. Quantitation of skeletal-muscle necrosis in a model compartment syndrome. *J Bone Joint Surg Am.*, 1981, 63(4), 631-6.

[31] Heppenstall, RB; Sapega, AA; Scott, R; Shenton, D; Park, YS; Maris, J; Chance, B. The compartment syndrome: an experimental and clinical study of muscular energy metabolism using phosphorus nuclear magnetic resonance spectroscopy. *Clin Orthop Relat Res*. 1988, 226, 138–155.

[32] Heppenstall, RB; Scott, R; Sapega, A; Park, YS; Chance, B. A comparative study of the tolerance of skeletal muscle to ischemia: tourniquet application compared with acute compartment syndrome. *J Bone Joint Surg Am*. 1986, 68, 820–828.

[33] Heppenstall, RB; Sapega, AA; Izant, T; Fallon, R; Shenton, D; Park, YS; Chance, B. Compartment syndrome: a quantitative study of high-energy phosphorus compounds using 31P-magnetic resonance spectroscopy. *J Trauma.*, 1989, 29, 1113–1119.

[34] Vaillancourt, C; Shrier, I; Vandal, A; et al. Acute compartment syndrome: how long before muscle necrosis occurs? *CJEM*. 2004, 6(3), 147-54.

[35] Zweifach, SS; Hargens, AR; Evans, KL; et al. Skeletal muscle necrosis in pressurized compartments associated with hemorrhagic hypotension. *J Trauma*. 1980, 20(11), 941-7.

[36] Heckman, MM; Whitesides, TE; Grewe, SR; et al. Histologic determination of the ischemic threshold of muscle in the canine compartment syndrome model. *J Orthop Trauma.*, 1993, 7(3), 199-210.

[37] Odland, R; Schmidt, AH; Hunter, B; et al. Use of tissue ultrafiltration for treatment of compartment syndrome: a pilot study using porcine hindlimbs. *J Orthop Trauma.*, 2005, 19(4), 267-75.

[38] Shuler, FD; Dietz, MJ. Physicians' ability to manually detect isolated elevations in leg intracompartmental pressure. *J Bone Joint Surg Am*. 2010, 92(2), 361-7.

[39] Mubarak, SJ; Hargens, AR; Owen, CA; et al. The wick catheter technique for measurement of intramuscular pressure: a new research and clinical tool. *J Bone Joint Surg Am*. 1976, 58, 1016-20.

[40] Mubarak, SJ; Owen, CA; Hargens, AR; et al., Acute compartment syndromes: diagnosis and treatment with the aid of the wick catheter. *J Bone Joint Surg Am.*, 1978, 60, 1091-5.

[41] Owen, CA; Mubarak, SJ; Hargens, AR; et al. Intramuscular pressures with limb compression: clarification of the pathogenesis of the drug-induced muscle-compartment syndrome. *New Engl J Med.*, 1979, 300(21), 1169-72.

[42] Matsen, FA; Winquist, RA; Krugmire, RB. Diagnosis and Management of Compartmental Syndromes. *J Bone Joint Surg Am.*, 1980, 62, 286–91.

[43] Heckman, MM; Whitesides, TE; Gewe, SR; et al. Compartment pressure in association with closed tibial fractures. The relationship between tissue pressure, compartment, and the distance from the site of the fracture. *J Bone Joint Surg Am.*, 1994, 76(9), 1285-92.

[44] McQueen, MM; Court-Brown, CM. Compartment monitoring in tibial fractures: the pressure threshold for decompression. *J Bone Joint Surg*, Br. 1996; 78-B: 99-104.

[45] Williams, PR; Russell, ID; Mintowt-Czyz, WJ. Compartment pressure monitoring: current UK orthopaedic practice. *Injury*, 1998, 29, 229-32.

[46] Gershuni, DH; Yaru, NC; Hargens, AR; et al. Ankle and Knee Position as a Factor Modifying Intracompartmental Pressure in the Human Leg. *J Bone Joint Surg Am.*, Dec 1984, 66(9),1415-20.

[47] Bernot, M; Gupta, R; Dobrasz, J; et al. The effect of antecedent ischemia on the tolerance of skeletal muscle to increased interstitial pressure. *J Orthop Trauma.*, 1996, 10, 555–9.

[48] Matsen, FA; Krugmire, RB; King, RV. Nicolas Andry Award. Increased tissue pressure and its effects on muscle oxygenation in level and elevated human limbs. *Clin Orthop Relat Res.*, 1979, (144), 311-20.

[49] Harrington, P; Bunola, J; Jennings, AJ; et al. Acute compartment syndrome masked by intravenous morphine from a patient controlled analgesia pump. *Injury*. 2000, 31, 387–9.

[50] O'Toole, RV; Whitney, A; Merchant, N; et al. Variation in diagnosis of compartment syndrome by surgeons treating tibial shaft fractures. *J Trauma*. 2009, 67, 735-41.

[51] McQueen, MM; Duckworth, AD; Aitken, SA; et al. The estimated sensitivity and specificity of compartment pressure monitoring for acute compartment syndrome. *J Bone Joint Surg Am.* 2013, 95(8), 673-7.

[52] Garr, JL; Gentilello, LM; Cole, PA; et al. Monitoring for compartmental syndrome using near-infrared spectroscopy: a noninvasive; continuous; transcutaneous monitoring technique. *J Trauma*. 1999, 46(4), 613-6.

[53] Mancini, DM; Bolinger, L; Li, H; Kendrick, K; Chance, B; Wilson, JR. Validation of near-infrared spectroscopy in humans. *J Appl Physiol.* 1994, 77, 2740–7.

[54] Scheeren, TW; Schober, P; Schwarte, LA. Monitoring tissue oxygenation by near infrared spectroscopy (NIRS): background and current applications. *J Clin Monit Comput.*, 2012, 26, 279-87.

[55] Pellicer, A; Bravo, Mdel C. Near-infrared spectroscopy: a methodology-focused review. *Semin Fetal Neonatal Med.*, 2011, 16(1), 42–9.

[56] Arbabi, S; Brundage, SI; Gentilello, LM. Near-infrared spectroscopy: a potential method for continuous, transcutaneous monitoring for compartmental syndrome in critically injured patients. *J Trauma.*, 1999, 47, 829-33.

[57] Gentilello, LM; Sanzone, A; Wang, L; et al. Near-infrared spectroscopy versus compartment pressure for the diagnosis of lower extremity compartmental syndrome using electromyography-determined measurements of neuromuscular function. *J Trauma.*, 2001, 51, 1-9.

[58] Giannotti, G; Cohn, SM; Brown, M; et al. Utility of near-infrared spectroscopy in the diagnosis of lower extremity compartment syndrome. *J Trauma.*, 2000, 48(3), 396-399.

[59] Shuler, MS; Reisman, WM; Kinsey, TL; et al. Correlation Between Muscle Oxygenation and Compartment Pressures in Acute Compartment Syndrome of the Leg. *J Bone Joint Surg Am.*, 2010, 92(4), 863-870.

[60] Bariteau, JT; Beutel, BG; Kamal, R; et al. The use of near-infrared spectrometry for the diagnosis of lower-extremity compartment syndrome. *Orthopedics.*, 2011, 34(3), 178.

[61] Shuler, MS; Reisman, WM; Whitesides, TE; et al. Near-Infrared Spectroscopy in Lower Extremity Trauma. *J Bone Joint Surg Am.*, 2009, 91(6), 1360-1368

[62] Klaus, S; Heringlake, M; Bahlmann, L. Bench-to-bedside review: microdialysis in intensive care medicine. *Crit Care.*, 2004, 8(5), 363-8.

[63] Hillered, L; Vespa, PM; Hovda, DA. Translational neurochemical research in acute human brain injury: the current status and potential future for cerebral microdialysis. *J Neurotrauma.*, 2005, 22(1), 3-41.

[64] Pojar, M; Mandak, J; Cibicek, N; et al. Peripheral tissue metabolism during off-pump versus on-pump coronary artery bypass graft surgery: the microdialysis study. *Eur J Cardiothorac Surg.*, 2008, 33(5), 899-905.

[65] Korth, U; Merkel, G; Fernandez, FF; et al. Tourniquet-induced changes of energy metabolism in human skeletal muscle monitored by microdialysis. *Anesthesiology.*, 2000, 93(6), 1407-12.

[66] Muller, M; Schmid, R; Nieszpaur-Los, M; et al. Key metabolite kinetics in human skeletal muscle during ischaemia and reperfusion: measurement by microdialysis. *Eur J Clin Invest.*, 1995, 25(8), 601-7.
[67] Doro, CJ; Sitzman, TJ; O'Toole, RV. Can intramuscular glucose diagnose compartment syndrome? *J Trauma Acute Care Surg.*, 2014, 76(2), 474-8.
[68] Elliot, K. Intramuscular PH: diagnosing acute compartment syndrome with confidence. 15th Annual EFFORT Congress. London, UK. June 2014.
[69] Odland, RM; Kizziar, R; Rheuark, D; et al. The effect of capillary ultra-filtration probes on skin flap edema. *Otolaryngol Head Neck Surg*. 2003, 128, 210–214.
[70] Odland, RM; Umeda, A; Stevens, S; et al. Reduction of tissue edema by microdialysis. *Arch Otolaryngol Head Neck Surg.*, 1995, 121, 662–666.
[71] Sutton, RL; Quist, H; Mathews, W; et al. Ultrafiltration reduces cerebral edema after traumatic brain injury. *Soc Neurosci Abstr.*, 1999, 25, 311
[72] Odland, RM; Schmidt, AH. Compartment syndrome ultrafiltration catheters: report of a clinical pilot study of a novel method for managing patients at risk of compartment syndrome. *J Orthop Trauma.*, 2011, 25(6), 358-365.
[73] Lawendy, AR; Bihari, A; Sanders, DW; et al. The severity of microvascular dysfunction due to compartment syndrome is diminished by the systemic application of CO-releasing molecule-3. *J Orthop Trauma.*, 2014, 28(11), e263-8.
[74] Kearns, SR; O'Briain, DE; Kelly, C; et al. N-acetylcysteine protects striated muscle in a model of compartment syndrome. *Clin Orthop Relat Res.*, 2010, 468, 2251-2259.
[75] Ott, MC; Scott, JR; Bihari, A; et al. Inhalation of carbon monoxide prevents liver injury and inflammation following hind limb ischemia/reperfusion. *FASEB J.*, 2005, 19, 106–108.
[76] Scott, JR; Cukiernik, MA; Ott, MC; et al. Low-dose inhaled carbon monoxide attenuates the remote intestinal inflammatory response elicited by hindlimb ischemia-reperfusion. *Am J Physiol Gastrointest Liver Physiol.*, 2009, 296, G9–G14.
[77] Nakao, A; Kimizuka, K; Stolz, DB; et al. Carbon monoxide inhalation protects rat intestinal grafts from ischemia/reperfusion injury. *Am J Pathol.*, 2003, 163, 1587–1598.

[78] Motterlini, R; Clark, JE; Foresti, R; et al. Carbon monoxide-releasing molecules: characterization of biochemical and vascular activities. *Circ Res*. 2002, 90, E17–E24.

[79] Motterlini, R; Otterbein, LE. The therapeutic potential of carbon monoxide. *Nat Rev Drug Discov*., 2010, 9, 728–743.

In: Compartment Syndrome
Editor: Anna P. Henderson

ISBN: 978-1-63482-831-4

Chapter 2

The Role of Anesthesia in the Prevention and Management of Compartment Syndrome

***P. Fennessy*[1*] *and S. Crowe*[2]**

[1]MB BCh BAO, MCAI, Adelaide & Meath National Children's Hospital, N.U.I.G., Dublin, Ireland

[2] MB BCh BAO, FFARCSI, Our Lady's Children's Hospital Crumlin, T.C.D. , Dublin, Ireland

Abstract

Compartment Syndrome (CS) may develop following substantial injury to the muscles of the leg or arm. This injury may be related to recent surgery or may follow a crush or direct blunt trauma. Anesthesia may influence the development through the use of regional anesthesia, optimum blood pressure control and oxygen delivery, and tailored analgesia in the peri-operative period.

This chapter reviews the evidence relevant to how the anesthesiologist can influence the genesis of compartment syndrome. It provides support for best anesthesia practice in an effort to avoid this complication which may have serious adverse effects for the patient. The authors provide a structure which facilitates rapid and frequent evaluation

[*] Corresponding author: paulfeno@hotmail.com

of compartment pressures post-operatively, and discusses the management of CS after it has become established in the injured limb.

The Pathogenesis of Compartment Syndrome

The development of compartment syndrome (CS) is due to a complex interplay between perfusion of the tissues, oxygen delivery at microvascular level, venous drainage of the tissues, and tissue oedema. Other factors contributing to the development of this complication include preexisting vital organ dysfunction, intra-operative events such as hemorrhage and transfusion, and peri-operative hemodynamic instability due to hypovolemia or sepsis.

Tissue hypoxia stimulates complex reactions between cellular and humoral mediators such as cytokines, kinins and complement. These mediators commence more interactions which result in generalized endothelial injury leading to a diffuse inflammatory response. This inflammatory response plays an important role in the evolution of tissue oedema, perfusion deficiency and compartment syndrome. During periods of critical hypoperfusion, the vital organs are protected at the cost of the peripheral microcirculation. This may explain why CS may develop in the absence of deterioration of cerebral, renal or coronary perfusion. Previous studies have suggested that maintenance of peripheral tissue perfusion in the first 8-12 hours post-operatively reduces the incidence of organ dysfunction and operative mortality [1]. Additional damage through surgical insult or direct trauma causes cell damage and tissue oedema, which further compromises the blood supply into the cells. The presence of oedema reduces the capacity for venous drainage within the muscle compartment, and the resulting back pressure exacerbates the existing hypoperfusion. This spiral of increasing oedema leading to increasing congestion produces the clinical picture of acute ischemia of the muscles, and necrosis if left unchecked. Given the potential for anesthesia care to influence tissue perfusion and oxygenation, it is clear there is a possible role in preventing the onset of this serious complication [2].

Contribution of Anesthesia to Compartment Syndrome

CS is most commonly secondary to trauma of the arm or leg. However a number of iatrogenic causes are recognised many of which the anesthetist may be implicated [3].

Patient Positioning

Malpositioning of patients for surgery is a well documented iatrogenic cause of CS. The position of the patient on the operating table, the duration of direct pressure on muscle compartments during surgery and the height of the muscle in relation to the heart are among factors suggested as being important in the development of CS. A number of case reports have shown that prolonged lithotomy position can lead to the development of CS [4, 5, 6]. This position is most commonly used in urological, colorectal and gynaecological procedures.

Table 1. [7]

Risk Factors for Development of Compartment Syndrome in Litotomy position:
Increased body mass index
Diabetes mellitus
Peripheral vascular disease
Prolonged surgery > 5 hours
Legs positioned above the heart
Significant peri-operative blood loss
Hypotension
Muscular calves
Presence of concomitant external compression devices

The mechanism of ischaemia-perfusion may well play a role in this setting. Prolonged elevation with combined hypotension may lead to low grade calf-ischaemia. Reperfusion may then result in CS.

There has been debate over whether or not intermittent compression stockings increase the risk of CS in the lithotomy position [8]. A study published in Anesthesiology measured lower limb compartment pressures in the supine and lithotomy position with and without pneumatic compression devices [9]. The results demonstrated a significant increase in intracompartmental pressure during lithotomy position, while the use of intermittent compression stockings significantly reduced compartment pressures in both the lithotomy and supine positions. It must be noted however that this study was conducted on healthy awake volunteers. The use of pneumatic compression devices and their role in the development of CS remains debatable.

The Lloyd-Davis stirrups have been cited as causing reduced muscle perfusion, although there is a lack of evidence to support the use of foot or ankle stirrups instead of stirrups which support the lower leg. It has been shown that removing the limb from the lithotomy position results in a reduction of compartment pressure [10]. There may therefore be a role for removing the lower limbs from the lithotomy position intermittently during long procedures. Alternatively the use of hydraulic stirrups to vary leg position and height intra-operatively may reduce the risk of CS. [7]

Tourniquet Use and Compartment Syndrome

Tourniquet use is another iatrogenic etiology of CS with previous cases being described [11, 12]. Prolonged tourniquet time is associated with reperfusion injury and also lactate and potassium release [13]. Good communication between the surgeon and anesthetist is essential to identify those at risk of developing CS. Ideally a section specific to tourniquet pressure and anticipated tourniquet time should be incorporated into both Time Out and Sign Out sections of the WHO Surgical Safety Checklist. The NHS have incorporated a section during Time Out regarding specific equipment requirements.

The safest tourniquet pressure is the lowest pressure which will stop the flow of arterial blood past the tourniquet. This should be based on the limb occlusion pressure (LOP), which can be measured by some tourniquet systems automatically. The relatively new concept of internal tourniquets allows the non-surgical areas of the limb to be perfused intra-operatively thus reducing overall tissue ischaemia.

During long cases the tourniquet should be released for intermittent reperfusion [3]. This is known as tourniquet downtime technique. There are no set guidelines regarding tourniquet deflation and re-inflation cycles but the anesthetist should inform the surgeon if the tourniquet time exceeds 120 minutes [14].

Extravasation of Solutions

Extravasation of solutions, especially contrast media, may cause severe pain on injection, or may be asymptomatic. Automated delivery systems used for contrast medium in CT scanning may cause problems [15]. Cases of CS have been reported in septic neonates following large fluid resuscitation [16, 17], with the use of intravenous mannitol [18, 19], and the administration of medications and fluids through intraosseous needles employed during cardiopulmonary resuscitation in both adults and children [20].

Table 2.

Risk of Compartment Syndrome with Tissue Extravasation:
• Neonate resuscitation
• Administration of IV contrast media
• Intraosseus needles
• Mannitol administration
• Pressurized delivery systems

Patient Monitoring

Monitoring systems, including non-invasive blood pressure (NIBP) and arterial lines, have been associated with CS [21]. Frequency of cuff cycling, excessive cuff pressures and firm application of the deflated cuff are considered risk factors for the development of CS [22]. Arterial cannulation may lead to distal ischaemia secondary to intimal dissection, thrombus and also haematoma formation at time of insertion and removal [23, 24].

Evaluation and Monitoring of Compartment Pressures and Signs of Compartment Syndrome

Diagnosis has historically been based clinically. A history of the patients subjective symptoms should be elicited, a targeted physical examination performed and the trend in patient analgesic requirements reviewed.

Clinical signs of CS include pain out of proportion to the injury exacerbated on passive stretching of the muscles, swelling, sensory disturbance, motor disturbance and pulselessness. These signs may present late and alone have a low sensitivity for diagnosis. These signs are more useful in their absence for excluding CS than their presence in diagnosis [25].

Table 3.

Monitoring Modalities:
• Compartmental pressure monitoring - Intermittent vs continuous • Near-infrared spectroscopy • Imaging - MRI - Pulse phase-locked loop ultrasound - Infrared imaging • Serum creatinine phosphokinase • Myoglobinuria

Compartmental pressure monitoring is a useful adjunct in the diagnosis of CS. Normal compartmental pressure is <10-12 mmHg [26]. Different absolute compartmental pressures for diagnosing CS have been suggested. However it is the compartmental perfusion pressure, DeltaP (difference between diastolic arterial pressure and compartmental pressure) that is deemed more important for diagnosis. The most commonly cited perfusion pressure for diagnosis of CS is 30 mmHg [27]. Differential pressure (difference between mean arterial pressure and compartmental pressure) may be more accurate [28]. Needle manometers are cheap and easy to use while catheters are useful for continuous compartmental pressure monitoring [28]. Transducer tipped probes are rapidly responsive to changing pressures and highly accurate [29, 30]. They do not require a saline-column system. If CS is suspected all compartments within the limb should be measured [31]. Continuous pressure monitoring should be performed on the compartment with the highest initial reading [28].

The use of routine intracompartmental monitoring in those identified as high risk for developing CS may aid in earlier diagnosis and improvement in patient outcome [31]. Those patients at high risk include prolonged lithotomy position (> 5 hours) and prolonged tourniquet time as already discussed. Measurement of baseline compartment pressures in these patients for comparison post-operatively may be beneficial [32].

It is important to observe the trend in compartmental pressures over time as opposed to one single reading. The use of transducer tipped catheter for continuous monitoring would allow for trend observations without subjecting the patient to repeated needle manometer readings. If compartment pressures are seen to be increasing the patient should be kept fasted post-operatively until improvement or a diagnosis of CS is made as urgent fasciotomy may be indicated.

Pre-operative diastolic blood pressure (DBP) is a good indicator for post-operative DBP, whereas there is a significant reduction in DBP intra-operatively secondary to anesthesia [33]. The implication of this is that the DeltaP (DBP minus compartmental pressure) will be lower intra-operatively as compared to post-operatively, thus affecting management decisions. This is another reason to monitor the trend in compartment pressures over time.

Near-infrared spectroscopy (NIRS) has a role in monitoring for compartmental ischaemia [34]. It directly measures tissue hypoxia. Muscle oxyhaemoglobin levels measured by NIRS reflect compartment pressure, perfusion pressure and myoneural function [35]. It is a non-invasive investigation and can be used continuously. It is however expensive and only measures to a limited depth. A recent study demonstrated no significant relationship between tissue oxygenation measured by NIRS and compartmental pressures [36]. It suggested that NIRS is not a reliable tool in the diagnosis of CS.

The use of imaging in CS is under evaluation. MRI can demonstrate established CS but is not useful in diagnosing evolving CS [31]. Pulse phase-locked loop ultrasound can analyze fascial displacement waveforms [37]. These correspond to arterial pulsations and change with increased compartmental pressure. Infrared imaging may also play a role in early diagnosis of CS by detecting discrepancies in surface temperature between distal and proximal parts of the injured limb [38]. Infrared imaging has the benefit of being portable and non-invasive.

Serum creatinine phosphokinase and myoglobinuria may be used as indicators for CS. They may be useful when the clinical picture is not clear but are not helpful for early diagnosis.

While diagnosis may be difficult, a delay in diagnosis can result in severe functional morbidity for the patient. A number of factors can lead to such a delay. It is therefore important to have a high index of suspicion in those at risk of developing CS.

In the intensive care setting an increase in analgesic or sedation requirements may be the only indicator of impending CS development.

Anesthetic-related factors remain a controversial topic that has been widely debated.

Table 4. [26]

Causes for Delay in Diagnosis of Compartment Syndrome:

- Patient-related
  - Extremes of age
  - Lack of awareness/confusion
  - Polytrauma
  - Concomitant nerve injury
  - Misdiagnosis of DVT
  - Spinal cord injury
- Critical care-related
  - Sedation/analgesia
- Anesthesia-related
  - Recovery from general anesthesia
  - Regional anesthesia
  - Analgesia (PCA)
- Other
  - Reliance on clinical signs

Anesthetic Considerations and Compartment Syndrome

General Anesthesia

Patients recovering from general anesthesia may have difficulty expressing their pain due to ongoing sedation. This may lead to a delay in diagnosis and functionally a worse outcome. In those patients identified to be at risk of developing CS, the use of short acting anesthetic agents may be of benefit. The inhalational anesthetic agent desflurane has a faster offset as compared to sevoflurane due to its lower blood:gas partition coefficient.

For total intravenous anesthesia (TIVA), using a combination of propofol and remifentanil infusions would also lead to a more rapid recovery. Remifentanil has an extremely short half-life (10 minutes) whereas propofol has a much longer elimination half-life (5-12 hours). The use of remifentanil would allow less propofol to be used and hence a more rapid awakening time.

Remifentanil is also a potent analgesic and would aid intra-operative pain control.

Analgesia

Different analgesia modalities have been implicated in delay in diagnosing CS. The symptoms of CS are more difficult to assess in the context of reduced consciousness. Analgesic techniques, which rely on the interruption of sensation, can reduce the incidence of self-report for increasing pain or paraesthesia.

The use of non-sedating analgesic agents avoids masking of the symptoms of CS. A sedation scale e.g. the Ramsay sedation score, should be used in combination with a validated pain assessment scale. If the patient gives a low pain score in association with a high sedation score, a greater index of suspicion for CS is warranted. An objective pain score will also allow the trend in patient pain to be monitored.

Patient-controlled analgesia (PCA) with morphine has been associated with a delay in diagnosis [39]. One study favoured intermittent IM morphine injections over PCA [40]. It was felt however that this was due to increased interaction between the patient and nursing staff. When using PCA in those at risk of CS a more conservative hourly bolus limit could aid earlier detection of impending CS [41]. It is important that nursing staff observe the trend in patient analgesic requirements. This can be easily monitored via the PCA pump as both the number of attempts and volume of morphine received by the patient are recorded.

Regional Anesthesia

The use of regional anesthesia in those at risk of CS is controversial due to its association with delay in diagnosis [42]. This association has largely been based on case reports [43]. However no randomized-controlled trials have been performed comparing outcomes in patients who developed CS in those who received regional anesthesia and those who did not [44].

Some regional anesthetic techniques have been implicated in delaying diagnosis of CS. The use of intravenous regional anaesthesia (IVRA) however has been the only form of regional anaesthesia that has been directly implicated in causing CS [44]. This may be secondary to the use of double tourniquets or injection of a volume of local anesthetic into a closed compartment [45]. One study however has shown that in the nontraumatic limb, simulated IVRA with normal saline did not increase intracompartmental pressures [46].

Neuraxial blockade has been implicated in delaying diagnosis of CS [43]. However there have been no case reports of single shot spinal or epidural anesthesia resulting in such a delay [44]. While continuous spinal anesthesia provides excellent intra-operative analgesia, it is not appropriate in the post-operative period as it causes a dense motor block and thus prevents the patient mobilizing and commencing rehabilitation. When performing spinal anesthesia it is important to remember that the use of adjuncts e.g. fentanyl, clonidine, morphine and neostigmine can prolong the analgesic effects of local anesthetics. Intrathecal morphine is particularly effective in prolonging the analgesic effect of spinal anesthesia. In this case lower dose local anesthetic should be administered.

Continuous epidural infusion provides excellent analgesia in the post-operative period. It has however been cited as a contributing factor in delayed diagnosis of CS. A review paper of paediatric patients in 2009 showed no clear evidence for such a delay in diagnosis [47]. The national paediatric epidural audit included 10,633 epidurals and described 4 incidents of CS, but diagnosis was not masked by epidural analgesia [48]. Mar et al., examined the effect of post-operative analgesia on diagnosis of lower limb CS [43]. 32 of the 35 patients had signs and symptoms of CS despite a working epidural. 18 of these patients also had documented breakthrough pain. 3 out of 35 patients did have a delay in diagnosis, however these patients had a dense motor and sensory block [49-51]. The use of lower local anesthetic concentrations with evolving practice in anesthesia has led to less motor and sensory block. Therefore patients are able to mobilize post-operatively and engage in physiotherapy [52]. There may be a role for intermittent cessation of the epidural infusion to assess for signs of CS. Analgesia can be achieved once again with a small bolus once satisfied that the symptoms are not present.

Peripheral nerve blockade may be performed for surgical anesthesia, usually upper limb, or for post-operative analgesia. Short acting local anesthetics such as lidocaine are less likely to obscure the signs of CS [44]. With the use of ultrasound guidance less local anesthetic is required and duration of blockade is shorter [53]. Post-operative analgesia can be achieved using long acting local anesthetics such a bupivicaine. Continuous peripheral nerve blockade is also extremely effective in providing post-operative analgesia [44]. Its use may be associated with fewer systemic side effects when compared with opioids. Once again intermittent cessation of local anesthetic infusion to assess for signs of CS may play a role.

Table 5. [44]

Regional Anesthesia Recommendations:
• Single shot spinal/epidural relatively safe
• Caution with continuous epidural if high risk of CS
• Single shot upper/lower limb peripheral nerve blocks relatively safe
• Caution with continuous peripheral nerve block if high risk of CS
• Use low dose/low concentration local anesthetics
• Use of short acting local anesthetics
• If using adjuncts decrease the local anesthetic dose
• Intermittent cessation of local anesthetic infusion
• U/S when performing blocks decreases dose of local anesthetic required
• Elective compartmental pressure monitoring with regional anesthesia

The Potential Influence of Anesthesia on the Outcome from Compartment Syndrome

Early diagnosis, prompt and appropriate treatment of CS can lead to a good functional outcome. Delayed diagnosis however is associated with significant disability, morbidity and mortality. Age > 50 years is a significant predictor of poor outcome [54]. This may be due to the likelihood that older patients undergo vascular procedures while trauma patients are younger and have a better overall outcome.

One study looked at the development of CS in the prolonged lithotomy position. 65 patients were identified. Of these 41.5% had permanent disability, 18.4% had significant muscle loss, 16.9% had foot drop or paraesthesia, death occurred in 6.1% and there was one case of renal failure secondary to rhabdomyolysis [7]. A delay in diagnosis occurred in 15 of the 65 patients and of those 15 patients 73.3% developed some form of permanent disability. This emphasises the need for early recognition and prompt treatment in this patient population.

Table 6.

Complications of Compartment Syndrome:
• Scarring secondary to fasciotomy
• Permanent disability
• Foot drop
• Paraesthesia
• Significant muscle loss
• Renal failure secondary to rhabdomyolysis
• Amputation
• Death in up to 15% of cases [54]
• Contractures

The mainstay of treatment of CS is surgical decompression by fasciotomy. Both the skin and fascia is incised to decrease tissue pressure, restore blood flow and minimize further tissue damage and related functional impairment. It is important to avoid hypotension intra-operatively and keep the limb at the level of the heart to optimize perfusion [26].

The anesthetist will have a major role in the peri-operative care of these CS patients. The anesthetist should be actively involved in the resuscitation of CS patients as they are at risk of developing systemic effects related to CS including rhabdomyolysis, renal failure, hyperkalaemia and cardiac instability. The anesthetist will also be engaged in analgesia management of these patients. Hyperbaric oxygen therapy has been advocated as an adjunct to fasciotomy in the treatment of CS [55, 56]. One double-blinded placebo-controlled trial randomly assigned patients with crush injuries to either hyperbaric oxygen therapy or normobaric oxygen therapy post-operatively. The group who received hyperbaric oxygen therapy had significantly improved wound healing and required fewer further surgical procedures such as skin flaps, grafts or amputation [57].

Table 7.

Suggested Benefits of Hyperbaric Oxygen Therapy:
• Increased tissue oxygenation
• Reduced oedema secondary to hyperoxia-induced vasospasm
• Protection from reperfusion injury and secondary ischaemia
• Antimicrobial effects

Mannitol may play a role in reducing the incidence of CS after limb revascularization. It acts as a free radical scavenger and also reduces oedema [26]. It may decrease the need for post-revascularization fasciotomy [58].

Conclusion

Compartment syndrome can be a devastating complication for the patient and is associated with significant morbidity and mortality. CS may have a higher incidence than is generally appreciated. We have reviewed the pathophysiology, risk factors, diagnosis, and management of acute compartment syndrome here.

It is important for the anesthetist to appreciate that it is not only the trauma patient at risk of developing CS. Factors such as patient positioning may be implicated as seen with the increased incidence of CS in patients undergoing radical cystectomy due to prolonged lithotomy position [7].

The anesthetist must tailor their anesthetic and analgesia plan to each individual patient, be aware of the recognised risk factors for a delay in diagnosis of CS while always having a low threshold for its potential diagnosis.

The cause of CS may be multifactorial but the anesthetist has a responsibility to the patient to recognise if they are at risk and communicate this to other healthcare providers, surgeons, critical care and nursing staff. This communication may be vital in leading to early diagnosis of the complication and better patient outcome.

References

[1] Kern JW, Shoemaker WC. Meta-analysis of hemodynamic optimization in high-risk patients. *Crit Care Med.* 2002 Aug;30(8):1686–92.

[2] Schober P, Schwarte LA. From system to organ to cell: oxygenation and perfusion measurement in anesthesia and critical care. J Clin Monit Comput. *Springer Netherlands;* 2012 Aug;26(4):255–65.

[3] Garner MR, Taylor SA, Gausden E, Lyden JP. Compartment syndrome: diagnosis, management, and unique concerns in the twenty-first century. *HSS J. Springer US;* 2014 Jul;10(2):143–52.

[4] Verdolin MH, Toth AS, Schroeder R. Bilateral lower extremity compartment syndromes following prolonged surgery in the low lithotomy position with serial compression stockings. *Anesthesiology.* 2000 Apr;92(4):1189–91.

[5] Mathews PV, Perry JJ, Murray PC. Compartment syndrome of the well leg as a result of the hemilithotomy position: a report of two cases and review of literature. *J Orthop Trauma.* 2001 Nov;15(8):580–3.

[6] Chow CE, Friedell ML, Freeland MB, Dejesus S. A pitfall of protracted surgery in the lithotomy Position: lower extremity compartment syndrome. *Am Surg.* 2007 Jan;73(1):19–21.

[7] Simms MS, Terry TR. Well leg compartment syndrome after pelvic and perineal surgery in the lithotomy position. *Postgrad Med J. The Fellowship of Postgraduate Medicine;* 2005 Aug;81(958):534–6.

[8] Cohen SA, Hurt WG. Compartment syndrome associated with lithotomy position and intermittent compression stockings. *Obstet Gynecol.* 2001 May;97(5 Pt 2):832–3.

[9] Pfeffer SD, Halliwill JR, Warner MA. Effects of lithotomy position and external compression on lower leg muscle compartment pressure. *Anesthesiology.* 2001 Sep;95(3):632–6.

[10] Chase J, Harford F, Pinzur MS, Zussman M. Intraoperative lower extremity compartment pressures in lithotomy-positioned patients. *Dis Colon Rectum.* 2000 May;43(5):678–80.

[11] Hirvensalo E, Tuominen H, Lapinsuo M, Heliö H. Compartment syndrome of the lower limb caused by a tourniquet: a report of two cases. *J Orthop Trauma.* 1992;6(4):469–72.

[12] Luk KD, Pun WK. Unrecognised compartment syndrome in a patient with tourniquet palsy. *J Bone Joint Surg Br.* 1987 Jan;69(1):97–9.

[13] Townsend HS, Goodman SB, Schurman DJ, Hackel A, Brock-Utne JG. Tourniquet release: systemic and metabolic effects. *Acta Anaesthesiol Scand.* 1996 Nov;40(10):1234–7.

[14] Murphy CG, Winter DC, Bouchier-Hayes DJ. Tourniquet injuries: pathogenesis and modalities for attenuation. *Acta Orthop Belg.* 2005 Dec;71(6):635–45.

[15] Bellin M-F, Jakobsen JA, Tomassin I, Thomsen HS, Morcos SK, Thomsen HS, et al. Contrast medium extravasation injury: guidelines for prevention and management. *European radiology.* 2002. pp. 2807–12.

[16] Christiansen SD, Desai NS, Pulito AR, Slack MR. Ischemic extremities due to compartment syndromes in a septic neonate. *J Pediatr Surg.* 1983 Oct;18(5):641–3.

[17] Talbot SG, Rogers GF. Pediatric compartment syndrome caused by intravenous infiltration. *Ann Plast Surg.* 2011 Nov;67(5):531–3.

[18] Edwards JJ, Samuels D, Fu ES. Forearm compartment syndrome from intravenous mannitol extravasation during general anesthesia. *Anesth Analg.* 2003 Jan;96(1):245–6–tableofcontents.

[19] Erickson BA, Yap RL, Pazona JF, Hartigan BJ, Smith ND. Mannitol extravasation during partial nephrectomy leading to forearm compartment syndrome. *Int Braz J Urol.* 2007 Jan;33(1):68–71–discussion71.

[20] Buck ML, Wiggins BS, Sesler JM. Intraosseous drug administration in children and adults during cardiopulmonary resuscitation. Ann Pharmacother. *SAGE Publications;* 2007 Oct;41(10):1679–86.

[21] Celoria G, Dawson JA, Teres D. Compartment syndrome in a patient monitored with an automated blood pressure cuff. *J Clin Monit.* 1987 Apr;3(2):139–41.

[22] Sutin KM, Longaker MT, Wahlander S, Kasabian AK, Capan LM. Acute biceps compartment syndrome associated with the use of a noninvasive blood pressure monitor. *Anesth Analg.* 1996 Dec;83(6):1345–6.

[23] Horlocker TT, Bishop AT. Compartment syndrome of the forearm and hand after brachial artery cannulation. *Anesth Analg.* 1995 Nov;81(5):1092–4.

[24] Qvist J, Peterfreund RA, Perlmutter GS. Transient compartment syndrome of the forearm after attempted radial artery cannulation. *Anesth Analg.* 1996 Jul;83(1):183–5.

[25] Ulmer T. The clinical diagnosis of compartment syndrome of the lower leg: are clinical findings predictive of the disorder? *J Orthop Trauma.* 2002 Sep;16(8):572–7.

[26] Farrow C, Bodenham A, Troxler M. Acute limb compartment syndromes. *Contin Educ Anaesth Crit Care Pain.* Oxford University Press; 2010 Nov 17;11(1):mkq041–28.

[27] Shadgan B, Menon M, O'Brien PJ, Reid WD. Diagnostic techniques in acute compartment syndrome of the leg. *J Orthop Trauma.* 2008 Sep;22(8):581-7.

[28] Elliott K, Johnstone AJ. Diagnosing acute compartment syndrome. *Journal of Bone and Joint* Vol 85 B No. 5 July 2003.

[29] Nakhostine M, Styf JR, van Leuven S, Hargens AR, Gershuni DH. Intramuscular pressure varies with depth. The tibialis anterior muscle studied in 12 volunteers. *Acta Orthop Scand.* 1993 Jun;64(3):377–81.

[30] Willy C, Gerngross H, Sterk J. Measurement of intracompartmental pressure with use of a new electronic transducer-tipped catheter system. *J Bone Joint Surg Am.* 1999 Feb;81(2):158–68.

[31] Köstler W, Strohm PC, Südkamp NP. Acute compartment syndrome of the limb. *Injury.* 2005 Aug;36(8):992–8.

[32] Prayson MJ, Chen JL, Hampers D, Vogt M, Fenwick J, Meredick R. Baseline compartment pressure measurements in isolated lower extremity fractures without clinical compartment syndrome. *J Trauma.* 2006 May;60(5):1037–40.

[33] Kakar S, Firoozabadi R, McKean J, Tornetta P. Diastolic blood pressure in patients with tibia fractures under anaesthesia: implications for the diagnosis of compartment syndrome. *J Orthop Trauma.* 2007 Feb;21(2):99–103.

[34] Gentilello LM, Sanzone A, Wang L, Liu PY, Robinson L. Near-infrared spectroscopy versus compartment pressure for the diagnosis of lower extremity compartmental syndrome using electromyography-determined measurements of neuromuscular function. *J Trauma.* 2001 Jul;51(1):1–8–discussion8–9.

[35] Garr JL, Gentilello LM, Cole PA, Mock CN, Matsen FA. Monitoring for compartmental syndrome using near-infrared spectroscopy: a noninvasive, continuous, transcutaneous monitoring technique. *J Trauma.* 1999 Apr;46(4):613–6–discussion617–8.

[36] Bariteau JT, Beutel BG, Kamal R, Hayda R, Born C. The use of near-infrared spectrometry for the diagnosis of lower-extremity compartment syndrome. *Orthopedics.* 2011 Mar;34(3):178.

[37] Wiemann JM, Ueno T, Leek BT, Yost WT, Schwartz AK, Hargens AR. Noninvasive measurements of intramuscular pressure using pulsed phase-locked loop ultrasound for detecting compartment syndromes: a preliminary report. *J Orthop Trauma.* 2006 Jul;20(7):458–63.

[38] Katz LM, Nauriyal V, Nagaraj S, Finch A, Pearlstein K, Szymanowski A, et al. Infrared imaging of trauma patients for detection of acute compartment syndrome of the leg. *Crit Care Med.* 2008 Jun;36(6):1756–61.

[39] Richards H, Langston A, Kulkarni R, Downes EM. Does patient controlled analgesia delay the diagnosis of compartment syndrome following intramedullary nailing of the tibia? *Injury.* 2004 Mar;35(3):296–8.

[40] Harrington P, Bunola J, Jennings AJ, Bush DJ, Smith RM. Acute compartment syndrome masked by intravenous morphine from a patient-controlled analgesia pump. *Injury.* 2000 Jun;31(5):387–9.

[41] Yang J, Cooper MG. Compartment syndrome and patient-controlled analgesia in children--analgesic complication or early warning system? *Anaesth Intensive Care.* 2010 Mar;38(2):359–63.

[42] Davis ET, Harris A, Keene D, Porter K, Manji M. The use of regional anaesthesia in patients at risk of acute compartment syndrome. *Injury.* 2006 Feb;37(2):128–33.

[43] Mar GJ, Barrington MJ, McGuirk BR. Acute compartment syndrome of the lower limb and the effect of postoperative analgesia on diagnosis. *Br J Anaesth.* Oxford University Press; 2009 Jan;102(1):3–11.

[44] Mannion S, Capdevila X. Acute compartment syndrome and the role of regional anesthesia. *Int Anesthesiol Clin.* 2010;48(4):85–105.

[45] Ananthanarayan C, Castro C, McKee N, Sakotic G. Compartment syndrome following intravenous regional anesthesia. *Can J Anaesth.* Springer-Verlag; 2000 Nov;47(11):1094–8.

[46] Mabee JR, Shean C, Orlinsky M, Androy L, Carter V. The effects of simulated Bier block IVRA on intracompartmental tissue pressure. *Acta Anaesthesiol Scand.* 1997 Feb;41(2):208–13.

[47] Johnson DJG, Chalkiadis GA. Does epidural analgesia delay the diagnosis of lower limb compartment syndrome in children? *Paediatr Anaesth.* Blackwell Publishing Ltd; 2009 Feb;19(2):83–91.

[48] Llewellyn N, Moriarty A. The national pediatric epidural audit. *Paediatr Anaesth.* Blackwell Publishing Ltd; 2007 Jun;17(6):520–33.

[49] Kontrobarsky Y, Love J. Gluteal compartment syndrome following epidural analgesic infusion with motor blockage. *Anaesth Intensive Care.* 1997 Dec;25(6):696–8.

[50] Somayaji HS, Hassan ANA, Reddy K, Heatley FW. Bilateral gluteal compartment syndrome after total hip arthroplasty under epidural anesthesia. *J Arthroplasty.* Elsevier; 2005 Dec;20(8):1081–3.

[51] Tang WM, Chiu KY. Silent compartment syndrome complicating total knee arthroplasty: continuous epidural anesthesia masked the pain. *J Arthroplasty.* 2000 Feb;15(2):241–3.

[52] Badner NH, Reid D, Sullivan P, Ganapathy S, Crosby ET, McKenna J, et al. Continuous epidural infusion of ropivacaine for the prevention of postoperative pain after major orthopaedic surgery: a dose-finding study. *Can J Anaesth.* Springer-Verlag; 1996 Jan;43(1):17–22.

[53] Harper GK, Stafford MA, Hill DA. Minimum volume of local anaesthetic required to surround each of the constituent nerves of the axillary brachial plexus, using ultrasound guidance: a pilot study. *Br J Anaesth.* 2010 May;104(5):633–6.

[54] Heemskerk J, Kitslaar P. Acute compartment syndrome of the lower leg: retrospective study on prevalence, technique, and outcome of fasciotomies. *World J Surg.* Springer-Verlag; 2003 Jun;27(6):744–7.

[55] Fitzpatrick DT, Murphy PT, Bryce M. Adjunctive treatment of compartment syndrome with hyperbaric oxygen. *Mil Med.* 1998 Aug;163(8):577–9.

[56] Wattel F, Mathieu D, Nevière R, Bocquillon N. Acute peripheral ischaemia and compartment syndromes: a role for hyperbaric oxygenation. *Anaesthesia.* 1998 May;53 Suppl 2:63–5.

[57] Bouachour G, Cronier P, Gouello JP, Toulemonde JL, Talha A, Alquier P. Hyperbaric oxygen therapy in the management of crush injuries: a randomized double-blind placebo-controlled clinical trial. *J Trauma.* 1996 Aug;41(2):333–9.

[58] Shah DM, Bock DE, Darling RC, Chang BB, Kupinski AM, Leather RP. Beneficial effects of hypertonic mannitol in acute ischemia--reperfusion injuries in humans. *Cardiovasc Surg.* 1996 Feb;4(1):97–100.

In: Compartment Syndrome
Editor: Anna P. Henderson

ISBN: 978-1-63482-831-4

Chapter 3

Compartment Pressure Monitoring

Rishi Dhir * ***and Matthew Barry***
Royal London Hospital, UK

Introduction

There are various underlying causes which initiate the sequence of events resulting in compartment syndrome including fractures, bleeding, tightly applied casts or extrinsic compression devices, burns and vigorous exercise. The common denominator appears to be an initial insult causing haemorrhage or oedema. This causes a rise in interstitial (tissue) fluid pressure in a closed osteofascial compartment (an anatomical space defined by rigid and unyielding boundaries). The result is vascular occlusion and subsequent reduced blood flow, the devastating sequelae of which are ischaemic necrosis of myoneural tissue and ultimate permanent contracture. This phenomenon was first described by Richard von Volkmann in 1881. [1]

The degree of functional loss depends upon how quickly surgical decompression of the involved compartment is performed. Decompression itself can carry considerable morbidity with risks of infection and difficulty in wound closure requiring further plastic surgical procedures, thus prompt and accurate diagnosis is vital.

* Corresponding author: rishimusic@hotmail.com; Rishi.Dhir@bartshealth.nhs.uk

Early clinical findings of raised intracompartmental pressure include swelling, palpable tenseness over a muscle compartment and pain out of proportion to the injury or on passive stretch of the muscles in the compartment. Later signs include reduced or absent sensation, muscle paresis and loss of pulses. However these can often be subjective. For example, pain or nerve injury may be initiated by the initial direct trauma rather than compartment syndrome. Also, except in the case of major arterial injury, pulses may often be palpable even when a compartment syndrome is present. In particular, patient groups such as children, those with impaired or absent consciousness and in whom clinical findings are equivocal can be very difficult to diagnose on clinical grounds and therefore having an objective test to aid diagnosis and subsequent surgical management of acute compartment syndrome is imperative.

Generic Principles of Monitoring

There are three essential components of conventional pressure monitoring systems. [2]

(1) A catheter tip placed at the tissue: fluid interface
(2) An external dome transducer
(3) Fluid-filled plastic tubing connecting the catheter tip to the transducer

Conventional systems were distinguished solely by the design of the catheter tip, as all use the same external dome transducer and connecting tubing. These catheter tips include wick catheters [1, 3], slit catheters [4], needle manometer [5] and continuous infusion catheters [6]. Most historical research has focused on advantages of one catheter tip over another, paying less attention to the other major shortcomings of the system; namely the external transducer and connecting tubing.

Problems associated with the external transducer include: difficulties in levelling the transducer dome with a catheter tip that is buried deep in the muscle; having to constantly re-level the transducer when the patient is moved and a prolonged set-up time.

Conversely, the connecting tubing also presents problems with numerous attachments, increasing the likelihood of breakdown and subsequent false pressure readings. Secondly, the presence of air bubbles can act as a dam in the tubing, preventing transmission of pressure from the muscle to transducer, leading to false low values and thirdly, a low frequency response capability. Newer techniques have focused on these areas [2].

Diagram of Generic Set Up

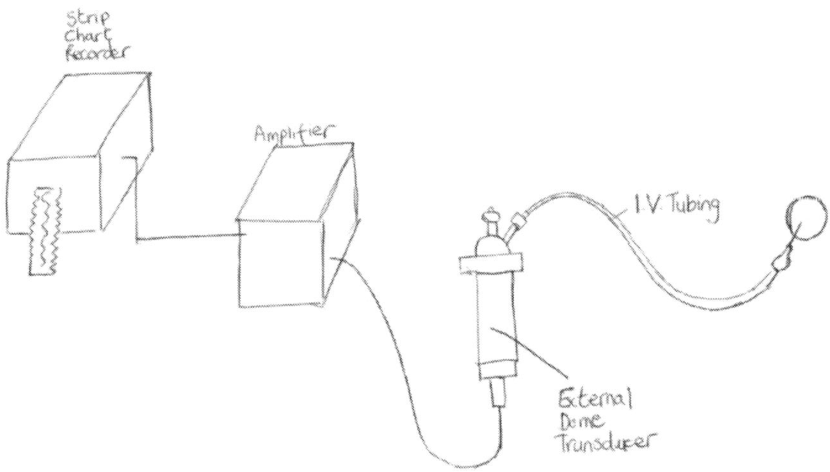

Adapted from McDermott et al., (1983) [2].

Classification

Compartment pressure monitors can broadly be subdivided into two main categories. Firstly, there are fluid-filled systems, consisting of fluid-filled tubing and a catheter tip connected to an extra-corporeal transducer. These may suffer from hydrostatic pressure artefacts and also the transducer must be at the level of the catheter. Secondly, the modern designs consist of transducer-tipped systems which incorporate the transducer into their design which is intracorporeal (within the muscle compartment) during measurements.

Several techniques have been used to prevent catheter occlusion by blood clots or soft tissue. The catheter tip can be open or closed and replaced by one or several side holes. Wick strands that extend from the catheter tip into the tissue [1] or slits at the catheter end [4] can be used. Protective sleeves around transducer tipped catheters (e.g. STIC catheter) [2] or injection or infusion of fluid to keep the tip open can be used. They can therefore be further subclassified into injection, infusion or non-infusion techniques and often they are a combination of these three.

1. Fluid-Filled Systems

A. Needle Manometer Technique

This is the most traditional technique, described by Landerer in 1884 and later modified for clinical use [5, 7, and 8]. It consists of a fluid-filled needle or pressure catheter, transducer, three-way stopcock, a syringe and manometer. It requires injection of free fluid and thus is an example of an injection technique.

It provides an assessment of *total tissue pressure* which is the sum of *solid tissue pressure* and *interstitial fluid pressure*. In this technique, the needle manometer system is closed by insertion of the needle into the muscle compartment. The external pressure is then slowly increased in this closed external system until motion of fluid or air meniscus into the compartment. The manometric pressure immediately before meniscal motion approximates the total tissue pressure. [7]

Techniques Measuring Total Tissue Pressure, Using the Needle Manometer System

It does however carry numerous problems. Saline injection creates non equilibrium conditions, as local oedema exists near the orifice of the needle and leads to falsely high tissue fluid pressures than usually recorded at equilibrium conditions. It measures total tissue pressure (sum of interstitial and solid tissue pressure) rather than interstitial fluid pressure in normal non oedematous tissue. It is also not possible to record dynamic pressures (during muscle contraction) or continuous long term recording and the needle tip is often occluded by tissue, rendering the technique insensitive or very slow to respond to changes in compartment pressures. To eliminate non-equilibrium conditions, the *interstitial fluid* must be measured directly, which has been experimentally determined by using implantable perforated spheres [10] subcutaneous fluid spaces [10] and the Wick catheter [1]. Of these only the latter allows immediate compartment pressure determination.

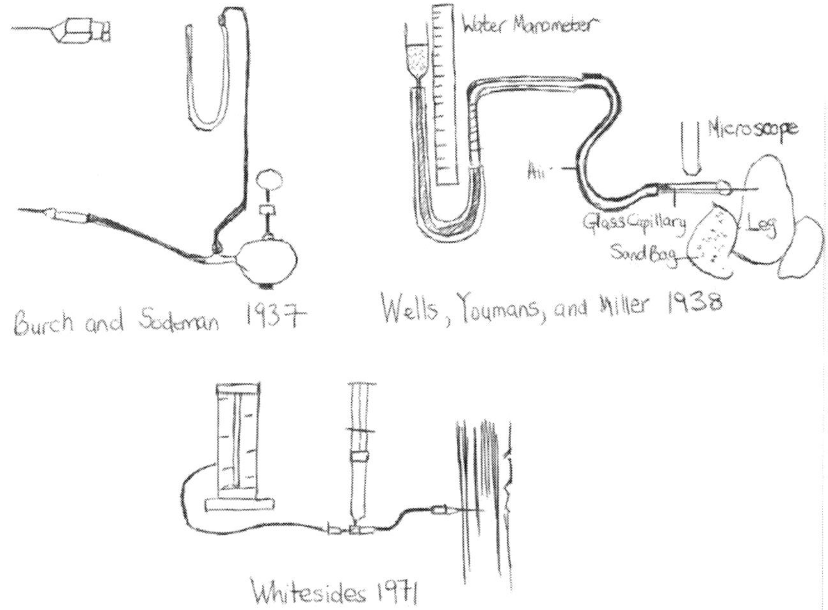

Adapted from Koman et al., (1981) [9].

B. Wick Catheter

First described by Scholander et al., (1968) [3] and later modified for clinical use [1, 11, 12], this popular technique seeks to eliminate conditions of non-equilibrium inherent in the needle manometer technique by directly measuring interstitial pressure. Its main design principle is to maintain catheter patency by placing microscopic fibres or filaments at the catheter tip [13]. It is an example of a non-infusion technique. Since most tissues have a sparsity of fluid, acute tissue fluid pressure studies depend on optimum contact between the free fluid in the tissue and saline within the measuring device. Wick fibres maintain this fluid continuity and increase the surface area of contact between the saline filled catheter and surrounding tissue fluids. It directly records tissue fluid pressure immediately following insertion as there is no fluid-gas interface present around the wick fibres and therefore, no capillarity. There is normally no osmotic effect across the tissue fluid-wick boundary as osmotically active particles such as red cells can pass freely between the wick fibres. Mubarak et al., [1, 12] showed in both human and canine studies that this technique was more accurate and reproducible than needle manometer and solid state pressure probes in measuring compartment pressures as it didn't cause disequilibrium conditions and was not dependent on the temperature or position in the compartment.

Catheter Construction

These wick fibres, which have varied in the literature from boiled cotton [3] to silk, dexon [1], nylon and other synthetic fibres, are pulled loosely into a plastic tube (catheter) by a monofilament tether, such as a 6/0 nylon suture, normally leaving 3-4mm of wick material outside the catheter tip. These wick fibres stop tissue plugging the catheter and should be frayed to maximise fluid contact area during subsequent placement in tissue. The catheter is flushed by heparinized saline before use which also helps prevent clot formation and prolong catheter use. The wick fibres should be packed loosely enough to allow good flow but not too loose to be pushed out by the flushing manoeuvre or pulled out by exercise. The catheter is then sterilised by ethylene oxide gas. [13].

Picture of wick catheter (photograph)

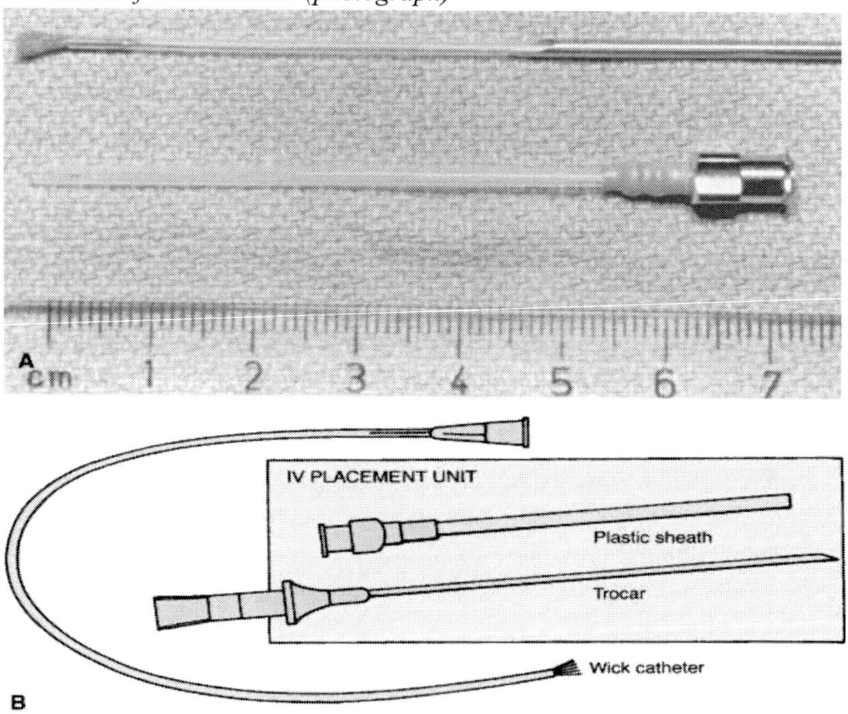

A: Photograph of Wick catheter inserted through trochar with plastic sheath below.
B: Diagram of plastic sheath, trocar and wick catheter.

Insertion of a Wick Catheter

Before insertion, the catheter is filled with sterile heparinised saline and connected via high pressure tubing and a three-way tap to a low volume-displacement pressure transducer. After calibrating the transducer to a given pressure range, the entire line is flushed with sterile saline to purge air bubbles from the pressure transducer dome to the wick fibres. The tip of the catheter is placed level with the site to be measured and the system is zeroed. It is important to check for small leaks in the saline-filled catheter as recording tissue fluid pressure accurately requires tight connections throughout the system. This can be done by clamping the catheter just proximal to the wick fibres and artificially raising and lowering pressure in the tubing and checking that recorded pressure remains constant. The catheter is the inserted into the muscle compartment of interest under local anaesthetic via a large bore needle (14 to 18 gauge) intravenous placement unit (inner steel trochar and plastic sheath) and the tissue fluid pressure is measured. This sequence of steps is essentially the same for insertion of other catheters such as the slit catheter. To reduce traumatic and inflammatory artefacts during pressure measurements, the wick tip is placed several centimetres from the site of local anaesthesia and skin puncture. Then, after the IV placement unit has penetrated the last barrier of tissue resistance (fascia for intramuscular measurements), the inner steel trocar is withdrawn slightly to a point just inside the plastic sheath during final insertion.

Typically wick catheters can record pressures for up to 8 hours and loosely fitting wick fibres optimise communication between tissue fluid and the recording system and lengthen the time over which measurements can be made. The technique does carry some problems, however. If the catheter is packed too tightly with wick fibres, its responsiveness to pressure alterations greatly decreases and after prolonged use, clotting usually develops at the wick: tissue interface, causing the catheter to act as a colloid osmometer and thus recording negative pressures. Therefore its use is limited to acute measurements of tissue fluid pressure, although recent changes in configuration and wick material have prolonged its recent use [13].

C. Slit Catheter

This uses a similar principle to the wick catheter to directly measure tissue fluid pressure and was first described by Rorabeck et al., [4]. It consists of 20 cm-long polyethylene tubing. The catheter tip in this case is cut so that five

30mm long symmetrical slits maintain patency without saline infusion, allowing free passage of interstitial fluid whilst preventing blockage of the tissues. It uses the same insertion technique as the wick catheter and is also a non-infusion technique.

Photo of Stryker slit catheter being inserted to measure the tibial compartment pressure

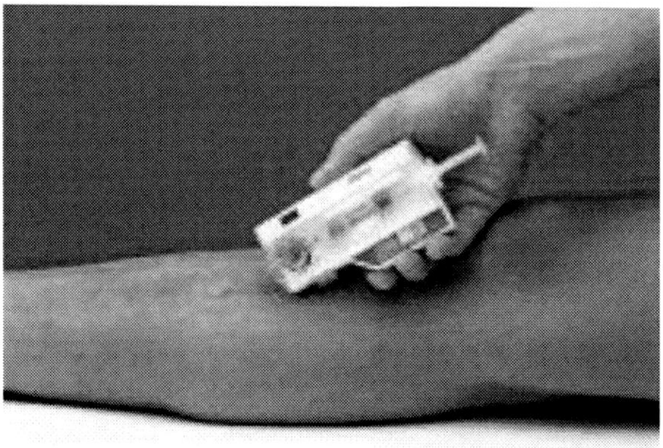

Comparative experimental studies of the wick and slit catheter techniques both in vitro and in vivo [14] were performed by inserting the catheters in saline or the anterolateral muscle compartment of human subjects, respectively and exposing them to extrinsic pressures via an inflatable pressure bag. These revealed that they are equally sensitive in recording tissue fluid pressures and also both avoid the non-equilibrium conditions inherent in the needle manometer technique. Its main advantages over the wick catheter include cheaper cost, greater responsiveness to changes in tissue fluid pressure especially during dynamic studies of muscle contraction, prolonged recording time due to the more open design of the catheter tip preventing blockage and the ability to break blood clots in vivo by applying pressure over the catheter tip. However air bubbles may be caught more easily in open ended catheters (slit) compared with catheters containing wick fibres and he slits can become distorted and occlude the tip of the catheter if used during exercise. The transducer must also be at the level of the catheter.

D. Myopress Catheter [13]

This is an example of a microcapillary infusion technique consisting of a 30cm catheter with four sideholes, which receives a nonconstant infusion during recordings. In vivo studies in exercising subjects [15] show that it compares favourably with non-infusion techniques such as the slit catheter in measuring dynamic compartment pressures during exercise.

It still suffers from the problems of hydrostatic artefacts because it consists of a saline-filled line connected between the subject and pressure transducer.

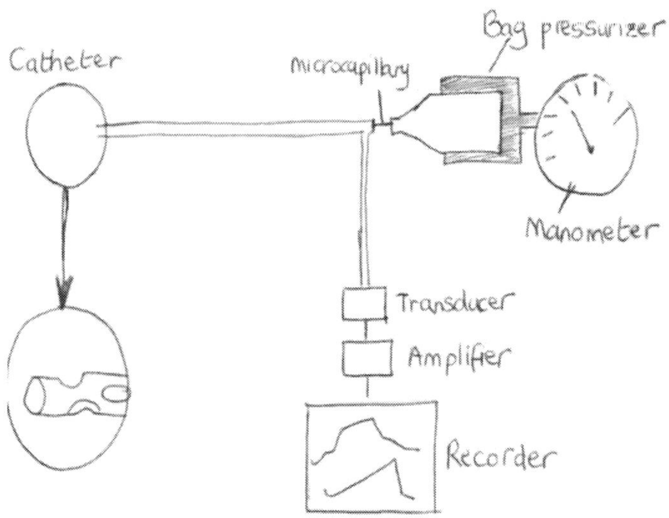

Schematic drawing of the Myopress system

Adapted from Hargens et al., [13].

2. Transducer-Tipped Systems

A. Fibre-Optic Catheter [16]

This is a transducer-tipped catheter. Studies have shown that in comparison with the slit catheter, it is as accurate for measuring tissue fluid pressures at rest but offers distinct advantages over conventional fluid-filled systems for measuring intramuscular pressures. This is due to a lack of hydrostatic pressure artefacts caused by limb position and to the lack of flushing requirements for long-term measurements [16]. Therefore it is much better at recording dynamic and continuous long-term measurements. It is, however, relatively large and must be attached to a saline-filled intracath sheath for tissue fluid measurements which causes patient discomfort compared with smaller catheter systems [17]. Other problems are that the large volume of the fibre optic system can cause piston effects during exercise (positive or negative intramuscular pressure artefacts during catheter movement) and heavy exercise or abnormal movements can cause the optical fibres to break [13]. Therefore this procedure is not commonly used in clinical applications.

Diagram of Fibre-Optic Catheter System

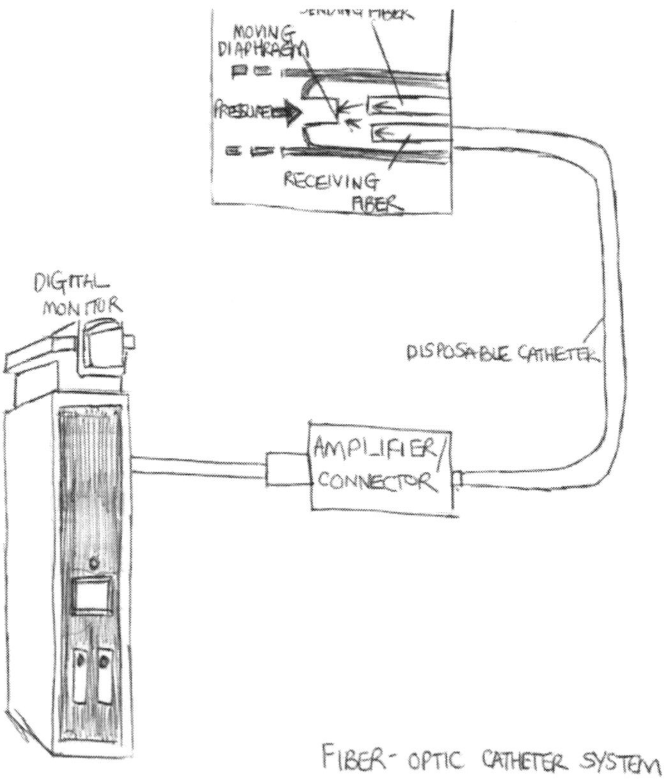

Adapted from Hargens et al., (1995) [13].

B. Electronic Transducer-Tipped Catheter

Experimental studies [17] have shown that they accurately measure intramuscular pressure, are small, minimally traumatic and easy to use. They are also highly sensitive, responding well to dynamic changes in pressure and also suitable for long-term recording with no loss of accuracy after twenty-one hours [17]. They also avoid the problems associated with fluid-filled catheters such as the wick catheter which can become blocked by clots and the slit catheter which requires numerous flushes for prolonged monitoring. They also, similar to the fibre optic catheter [16] don't suffer from movement artefacts during extreme muscle activity such as changes in patient position. However they are resistant to the dislocation and breakage of the inserted transducer tip catheter and electronic artefacts that the fibre-optic catheter suffers from during strong muscular activity therefore are more suitable for clinical applications.

Diagram of Electronic Transducer-Tipped Catheter [17]

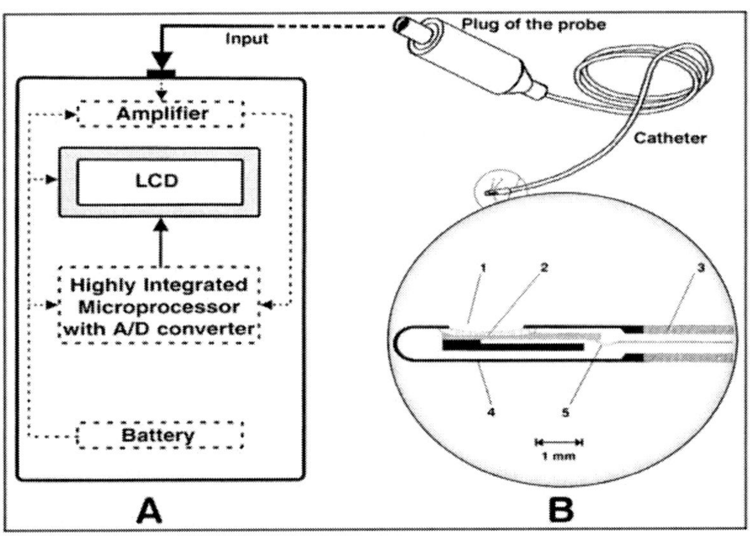

Diagram showing the components of the handheld device and electronic transducer tipped catheter.

A: The handheld device consists of an amplifier, a highly integrated microprocessor with an analogue to digital (A/D) converter, a nine-volt battery and liquid crystal display (LCD).

B: The magnified detail of the electronic transducer-tipped catheter (side view) shows the pressure-sensing mechanics of the catheter tip. An increase in tissue pressure causes a rise in the pressure of the surface of the piezoelectric crystal, resulting in changes in the electrical resistance. After amplification and conversion to digital signals, the pressure is immediately displayed on a liquid crystal-display monitor.
1 = small measuring window; 2 = unicrystalline piezo semiconductor with a chip; 3 = tip of the sixty-centimetre polyurethane catheter; 4 = stainless-steel housing and 5 = wires to the connector.

Conclusion

Compartment pressure monitoring provides a very useful method of helping to confirm the diagnosis of compartment syndrome, particularly in those cases or subjects where the clinical picture is equivocal. Traditional fluid-filled systems with the focus on the catheter tip such as the wick and slit catheter have mainly been used. However, these catheters are not suitable for high fidelity, dynamic studies of exertional compartment syndrome or long-term monitoring. The recent development of miniature transducer-tipped catheters also provides more artefact free readings which are suitable in dynamic pressure monitoring.

References

[1] Mubarak SJ, Hargens AR, Owen CA et al., (1976). The wick catheter technique for measurement of intramuscular pressure. *J. Bone and Joint Surg.*; 58- A (7): 1016-20

[2] McDermott AGP, Marble AE, Yabsley RH (1984). Monitoring acute compartmental pressures with the S.T.I.C. catheter. *Clin. Orthop* 192-8

[3] Scholander PF, Hargens AR, Miller SL. (1968). Negative pressure in the interstitial fluid of animals. *Science* 161: 3221-8

[4] Rorabeck CH, Castle GSP, Hardie R et al., (1981) Compartmental pressure measurements: An experimental investigation using the slit catheter. *J. Trauma* 21: 446-9

[5] Burch GE, Sodeman WA (1937). The estimation of the subcutaneous tissue pressure by a direct method. *J. Clin. Invest*; 16: 845-50

[6] Matsen FA, Winquist RA and Krugmire RB. (1980)Diagnosis and management of compartment syndromes. *J. Bone and Joint Surg.* 62-A: 286-91

[7] Wells HS, Youmans JB, Miller DG Jr. (1938) Tissue pressure (intracutaneous, subcutaneous and intramuscular) as related to venous pressure, capillary filtration and other factors. *J. Clin. Invest* 17: 489-99.

[8] Whitesides TE Jr, Haney TC, Morimoto K et al., (1975). Tissue pressure measurements as a determinant for thc need for fasciotomy. *Clin. Orthop.* 113: 43-51

[9] Koman A, Hardaker WT and Goldner JL. (1981) Wick catheter in evaluating and treating compartment syndromes. *Southern medical journal* 73 (3): 303-9.

[10] Guyton AC (1963). A concept of negative interstitial pressure based on pressures in implanted perforated capsules. *Circ. Res.* 12: 39-414.

[11] Snashall PD, Lucas J, Guz A et al. (1971). Measurements of interstitial 'fluid' pressure by means of a cotton wick in man and animals: an analysis of the origin of the pressure. *Clin. Sci.* 41: 35-53

[12] Mubarak SJ, Owen CA, Hargens AR et al., (1978) Acute compartment syndromes: Diagnosis and treatment with the aid of the wick catheter. *J. Bone and Joint Surg* 60-A (8): 1091-6

[13] Hargens AR, Ballard RE. (1995) Basic principles for measurement of intramuscular pressure. *Operative techniques in sports medicine* vol 3 (4); 237-42

[14] Shakespeare DT, Henderson NJ, Clough G (1982). The slit catheter: a comparison with the wick catheter in the measurement of compartment pressure. *Injury.* 13 (5): 404-8

[15] Styf JR, Crenshaw AG and Hargens AR. (1989) Intramuscular pressures during exercise: comparison of techniques with and without infusion. *Acta Orthop. Scand* 60 (5); 593-6

[16] Crenshaw AG, Styf JR, Mubarak DJ and Hargens AR. (1990) A new "transducer-tipped" fiber optic catheter for measuring intramuscular pressures. *J. Orthop. Res;* 8: 464-8

[17] Willy C and Sterk J (1999). Measurement of Intracompartmental Pressure with use of a new electronic transducer-tipped catheter system. *J. Bone and Joint Surg.*; 81-A (2): 158-68

In: Compartment Syndrome
Editor: Anna P. Henderson

ISBN: 978-1-63482-831-4

Chapter 4

Compartment Syndrome in Mangled Upper Extremity

***Marius Fodor*[1,*]*, Raluca Sobec*[2] *and Lucian Fodor*[2]**
[1]Department of General Surgery, Emergency District Hospital, Cluj-Napoca, Romania
[2]Department of Plastic and Reconstructive Surgery, Emergency District Hospital, Cluj- Napoca, Romania

Abstract

Acute limb compartment syndrome (LCS) is determined by edema and bleeding in a restrained muscle compartment limited by fascia and bone. LCS leads to muscle and nerve ischemia, threatening limb function and viability. The most frequent etiological factors are trauma and reperfusion, followed by acute arterial occlusion. Left untreated, LCS can result in muscle necrosis and limb loss and, in severe cases, renal impairment and even death. The mangled upper extremity is a limb with trauma involving bone, soft tissue, nerves and vessels. Arterial and venous injuries are present in 42% of patients with severe upper extremity trauma. Emergency reconstruction of the upper extremity after severe trauma has a better outcome than late reconstruction. Treatment includes tissue debridement, irrigation of traumatized tissue, stable fixation of bone, revascularization, nerve repair and coverage of soft tissue. The sequence of restoration of these anatomical structures depends

[*] Corresponding author: Email: drfodor@yahoo.com

on the ischemia time and the severity of injury. Preventing or treating compartment syndrome in severe cases is a cornerstone of the beginning of treatment. A gradual approach to the severe mangled extremity is further detailed.

Compartment syndrome (CS) represents increased pressure of interstitial fluid inside an unexpansible osseofascial space, leading to alteration of microcirculation and myoneural necrosis. The main signs of CS are: inappropriate pain associated with injury, passive movement of limb associated with pain and palpation of compartment under tension. CS does not have a direct relation to arterial pulses: the absence of pulses is a late sign of CS and the presence of pulses could be associated with CS. The intracompartmental pressure can be as high as 50mmHg in CS [1-3].

CS associated with a mangled extremity is a particular condition. The term "mangled" is used for injury of a limb (avulsion, crushing or cutting) leading to anatomical deterioration of the extremity. Usually, the mangled extremity is a result of major trauma and associates important injuries of the following tissues: muscles, vessels, nerves, and bones [4]. Also, the word, "mangled", is used to define severe crush injuries, blast trauma and major extremity amputations.

In some cases, the mangled extremity is a part of complex life-threatening trauma. In this situation, the extremity trauma must be preceded by resuscitation and treatment of all life-threatening lesions, following the principle of "life before limb" [5].

Whether to amputate or to salvage the mangled extremity after high-energy trauma is a difficult decision to make. Trauma scales for extremity injury have been developed which evaluate the chance of limb salvage: Mangled Extremity Severity Score (MESS), Predictive Salvage Index (PSI), Limb Salvage Index (LSI), and Mangled Extremity Syndrome Index (MESI). The most common and accepted evaluation system is MESS and includes four parameters: age, shock, limb ischemia, skeletal/soft tissue trauma [6]. Each parameter is associated with points:

1) Age: below 30 years (0 points), 30-50 years (1 point), above 50 years (2 points)
2) Shock: systolic blood pressure above 90mmHg (0 points), temporary hypotension (1 point), persistent hypotension (2 points)

3) Limb ischemia: perfusion within normal limits (1 point); pulse loss with paresthesia and low capillary refill (2 points); insensitive, paralyzed and cool limb (3 points)
4) Skeletal/soft tissue lesions: low energy trauma (e.g. single bone fracture) (1 point); medium energy trauma (e.g. associated bone fractures) (2 points); high energy trauma (e.g. car crash injuries) (3 points); very high energy trauma (e.g. limb trauma with important contamination) (4 points)

The score is multiplied by two when the ischemic time for the limb is over six hours. MESS above 7 is correlated with a high rate of extremity amputation. This is not a rule - the final decision (salvage or amputation of the limb) is taken in each particular trauma situation [7-9].

Frequency and Causes for Mangled Upper Extremity

Extremity trauma in army conflicts (e.g. Iraq and Afghanistan) has been reported to be as high as 54%, and the rate of mangled limbs varies from 23-39%, depending on the severity of the lesions [10, 11]. The frequency of vascular injuries related to mangled extremities is 10-48% and the amputation rate in distal parts of the limb can be up to 85%. The mortality rate of patients with complex extremity injuries is 10% in army conflicts, comparing with civilian trauma where it is very rare [10, 11]. Death caused by an isolated limb lesion in civilian practice is encountered with associated morbidities in the elderly. When the mangled limb is part of multiple organ trauma, mortality is significantly high [12].

The causes of mangled extremity are related to high energy trauma of the patient, as seen in the following situations:

- motor vehicle crashes at high speed
- earthquakes with crush trauma
- complex lesions in bombs, munitions or mine explosions during war or terrorist attack [13, 14].

The mangled upper extremity is associated particularly with vehicle rollover accidents.

The principle of "keep your arms inside a moving vehicle" is forgotten by most traumatized patients. The amputation rate is 42% when the upper limb complex trauma is related to important soft tissue loss, multiple bone fractures and extensive vascular lesions [15].

Vascular lesions of the upper extremities are reported to vary from 3.3% to 3.7% in civilian trauma. Penetration injuries are present in 90% of cases and blunt injury in 10%.

The overall rate of amputation of the mangled extremity is 0-3.7% of cases. A penetrating lesion of the subclavian artery is related to significant mortality rates (5.2-39%). Blunt vascular injuries are correlated with higher amputation rates than penetration injuries [16].

Important Anatomy of the Upper Extremity

The upper extremity has three anatomical parts: upper arm, forearm and hand.

The upper arm has two different compartments: the anterior and the posterior but, according to some authors, a third compartment has been described as a component part of the upper arm – the deltoid compartment [17].

The *anterior upper arm compartment* is bounded laterally, anteriorly and medially by the brachial fascia and posteriorly by the humerus, medial and lateral intermuscular septa. It encompasses the coracobrachialis, biceps and the brachialis muscles, the median, ulnar, musculocutaneous nerve and the brachial artery.

The *posterior upper arm compartment* comprises the triceps brachialis muscle, radial nerve and deep brachial artery.

The forearm is divided into three important compartments, due to deep forearm fascia, interosseous membrane and fibrous intermuscular septa: the anterior compartment, which holds the wrist and finger flexors; the posterior compartment, where the wrist and finger extensors are located; and the mobile wad [18].

The *anterior forearm compartment* is bounded laterally, anteriorly and medially by the antebrachial fascia and, at the posterior side, by the lateral intermuscular septa, the radius, the interosseous membrane, the ulna and the medial intermuscular septa, while the *posterior forearm compartment* is defined anteriorly by the same structures as the posterior side of the anterior compartment and laterally, posteriorly and medially by the antebrachial fascia.

The *anterior forearm compartment* includes superficial and deep flexor compartments. The superficial flexor compartment includes pronator teres, flexor carpi radialis, palmaris longus, flexor digitorum superficialis, and flexor carpi ulnaris muscles, while the deep flexor compartment refers to flexor digitorum profundus, flexor pollicis longus and pronator quadratus muscles. The most important neuro-vascular structures that pass the anterior forearm compartment are: the brachial artery (in the proximal part) which divides into the radial and ulnar arteries, ulnar and median nerves, anterior interosseous nerve and superficial branch of the radial nerve.

The *posterior forearm compartment*, also known as the extensor compartment, encompasses the extensor digitorum, extensor digiti minimi, extensor carpi ulnaris and anconeus muscle situated superficially and abductor pollicis longus, extensor pollicis longus, extensor pollicis brevis, extensor indicis and supinator muscles situated deeper [18]. The posterior interosseous nerve passes through this compartment.

The mobile wad, limited by the radius, intermuscular septum and antebrachial fascia, includes the brachioradialis muscle, extensor carpi radialis brevis and extensor carpi radialis longus muscles and is crossed by the superficial branch of the radial nerve.

The hand is clinically divided into 12 compartments: the carpal and Guyon tunnels, the adductor compartment, thenar (abductor pollicis brevis, flexor pollicis brevis, opponens pollicis muscles and the flexor pollicis longus tendon passing by) and hypothenar compartments (abductor digiti minimi, flexor digiti minimi brevis, opponens digiti minimi muscles), three palmar and four dorsal interossei compartments. Cadaver studies on enclosed myofascial spaces in the hand have shown greater variability, and subcompartmentalization should be taken into account, as more than 50% of cases showed the presence of at least two compartments in the thenar or hypothenar eminences [19], although more recent cadaveric studies have shown that the intrinsic muscles of the hand are not completely surrounded by a fascia [20].

Clinical Signs of upper Extremity Compartment Syndrome

Clinical Signs

If obvious symptoms or signs of compartment syndrome in the upper extremity are present, fasciotomies are required and routine measurements of intracompartment pressure are not mandatory.

The presence of compartment syndrome and the need for fasciotomies are quite uncommon in the upper extremity, even in an busy level I trauma center [21]. Attention should be given to the arm compartment syndrome in a mangled upper extremity. Isolated arm compartment syndromes are very rare and the evaluation of an ipsilateral forearm for a possible compartment syndrome is advisable [21].

The clinical hallmark of limb compartment syndrome is the presence of pain disproportionate to the injury (in a conscious and aware patient). Also, the presence of the five Ps (pain, pallor, paresthesia, paralysis, pulselessness) are described for limb compartment syndrome.

Pain

The classical description of pain in an acute upper limb compartment syndrome is pain out of proportion to the injury, either at rest or during the stretch test, or at compression of the intracompartmental muscles [2, 22]. The pain is usually described as being different from the pain experienced with the trauma and is non-responsive to common analgesics.

Paresthesia and Paralysis

Paresthesia on the nerve territory that passes through the affected compartment is an impending early sign of nerve ischemia. If the ischemic process is allowed to proceed, anesthesia will occur, leading to paralysis at the end [1].

Pallor and Pulselessness

Clinically, the lack of a blood supply is defined by the presence of pallor. In an upper mangled extremity compartment syndrome, pallor is not a reliable sign. The absence of a pulse, if not correlated with direct arterial trauma, is a delayed sign in a compartment syndrome and predicts a bad prognosis [1]. The assessment of mangled upper extremity compartment syndrome differs according to the general condition of the patient, type of injury and other co-morbidities.

In **conscious patients**, the compartment syndrome diagnosis is based on the clinical features. The key symptoms and signs are: increasing and non-responsive to analgesics pain, sharp pain caused by the stretching test.

In **unconscious**, **sedated** patients or in the presence of another **sensory impairment** (central or peripheral nerve lesion), and based on the clinical findings (tenderness, swelling, bruising) and injury mechanism (e.g. high-energy trauma), suspicion of compartment syndrome might be raised. In these cases, ICP monitoring is important and helpful for an accurate diagnosis [22]. When suspicion of compartment syndrome is made in unconscious patients, side-by-side intracompartmental pressure measurement is recommended.

In **children**, upper extremity compartment syndrome is very rare but still a very serious and difficult to diagnose condition. Different studies have shown that the five Ps are inconsistent indicators for upper limb compartment syndrome in children. Increasing doses of analgesics are a possible sign of compartment syndrome development [5]. Other studies on upper extremity compartment syndrome in children reported pain and swelling as the most common presenting symptoms, while motor and sensory defects were not described very often [23]. Therefore, measuring the intracompartmental pressure is recommended in pediatric cases, when in doubt.

Intracompartmental Pressure Measurements for upper Extremity Compartment Syndrome

Intracompartmental pressure (ICP) measurement to define an upper limb compartment syndrome is not always necessary. The diagnosis is usually made clinically. ICP measurements are necessary in the following conditions:

- Unclear clinical signs of upper extremity compartment syndrome
- Children
- Unconsciousness patient
- Equivocal clinical signs and symptoms [1]
- Every doubtful case [22]

Reviewing the medical literature, many ICP measuring methods have been described: the infusion technique described by Whitesides et al., [24, 25], the wick catheter technique, Matsen's continuous infusion and monitoring, Weiner's catheter technique, Stryker ICP Monitor System [27]. A simple method to determine the intracompartmental pressure requires an arterial pressure monitoring device connected to a needle to be inserted in the compartment to be tested [26].

An intracompartmental pressure above 30-45mmHg is considered diagnostic for compartment syndrome [22] and requires fasciotomies. A high number of false-positive results have been reported in a traumatized limb for both ICP and the perfusion pressure (diastolic blood pressure − compartment pressure) [27]. Different experimental models have been developed and the accuracy of various methods of intracompartmental pressure measuring systems has been tested. In a study where the Stryker ICP Monitor System, an arterial line manometer, and the Whitesides method were evaluated, Boody and Wongworawat concluded that the arterial line manometer was the most accurate method, followed by the Stryker device [28].

Treatment of upper Extremity Compartment Syndrome

There are no specific guidelines for the treatment of compartment syndrome in the upper extremity, but there are some recommendations for particular situation. The British Medical Journal's Evidence Centre developed an algorithm for the management of acute compartment syndrome [29]. The steps of this algorithm are:

1) If the patient has an occlusive dressing:
   - first line treatment is to eliminate the compression caused by the dressing associated with supportive therapies (pain treatment, mannitol and intravenous hydration)
   - second line treatment is represented by fasciotomy and supportive therapies
   - third line treatment is amputation
2) If the patient does not have an occlusive dressing:
   - first line treatment is fasciotomy and supportive therapy
   - second line treatment is amputation

In both conditions, intravenous fluid treatment with urinary alkalinisation is indicated, if rhabdomyolysis is present.

The first step in treatment is to remove the compressive casts or splints overlying the anatomical area with possible increased ICP. A study developed on 26 dog limbs showed that removing the plaster reduced ICP by 65%, and cutting of padding resulted in an additional 20% decrease in ICP [30]. Most surgeons insist on continued limb evaluation for compartment syndrome differential diagnosis, even after elimination of tight casts. The upper limb should be placed at the heart level, in order to sustain compartment perfusion [1].

In cases of persistent acute compartment syndrome (ACS) after the above-mentioned maneuver, fasciotomy should be performed. Murphy made a first fascial decompression using a 3-6 inch incision on the antero-ulnar fascia for forearm compartment syndrome. Some authors have demonstrated that Jepson was the pioneer in fascial decompression, even if he published his techniques after Murphy [31]. It is useless to perform fasciotomy in cases of muscle death, due to crush syndrome. A more conservative approach is preferred until surgery can be performed in multiple trauma patients [32].

Mubarak and Hargens [33] recommend fasciotomy in the following cases:

1) ICP greater than 20mmHg associated with hypotension
2) ICP greater than 30mmHg in unconscious patients
3) Normal blood pressure but with compartment pressure greater than 30mmHg for more than eight hours

Fasciotomy should be performed with a large incision in order to totally decompress compartments with high pressure. In the forearm, volar and dorsal incisions are preferred to decompress all forearm compartments. In the hand, the carpal tunnel must be decompressed. Interosseus muscles could be released by two dorsal incision. Mid-lateral incisions are sufficient for digital decompression [34].

There is no consensus regarding the time of wound closure after fasciotomy, but primary wound closure is not commonly indicated. Mangled extremities are associated with multiple muscle involvement and often serial debridements are necessary. When feasible, preventing wound retraction should be performed but without any pressure on wound edges.

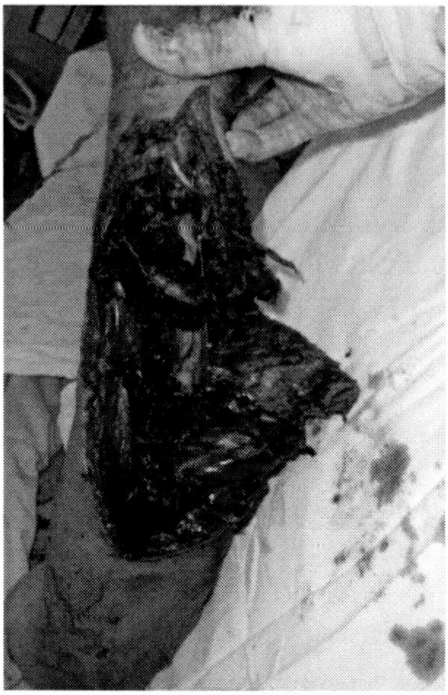

(a)

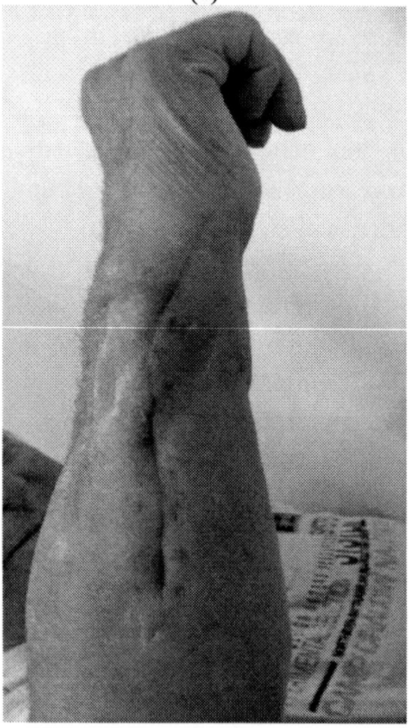

(b)

Figure 1. (Continued).

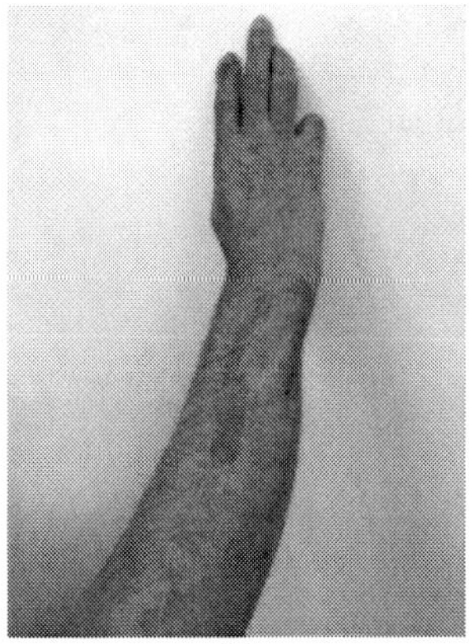

(c)

Figure 1. A. Mangled forearm after working accident. B. The wound was closed by delayed suture and skin graft. Finger flexion after bone stabilization and tendon repair. C. Extension lag on the 4th and 5th fingers; six months after the accident.

Among methods of closure reported, 59% of patients received delayed primary closure after fasciotomy, 15% had primary closure and 26% were treated by skin grafts [35]. Late closure of wounds after fasciotomy can be accomplished after repeat irrigation and debridement (Figure 1). Various surgical techniques can be used for skin closure: vacuum-assisted device, shoelace suturing techniques, skin graft (Figure 2) or flaps (Figure 3).

It is very important to perform the fasciotomy in a correct manner, thus avoiding the following pitfalls:

- The fascia should be completely incised, relieving swelling and tightness of the entire compartment
- The skin incision should be long enough to avoid compartment compression after the fasciotomy through a short skin incision [1]

The complications of fasciotomy are related to its delay rather than to the surgical act itself. Thus, muscle deterioration occurs within 2-4 hours after ischemia onset and becomes irreversible in 12 hours. Nerve lesions begin after 30 minutes of ischemia and become irreversible in days. About 68% of patients have normal functioning of the upper extremity, if the fasciotomy is done within 12 hours after acute onset of compartment syndrome. Complete functional restoration of the limb can be achieved if an urgent fasciotomy is performed in the first four hours [36].

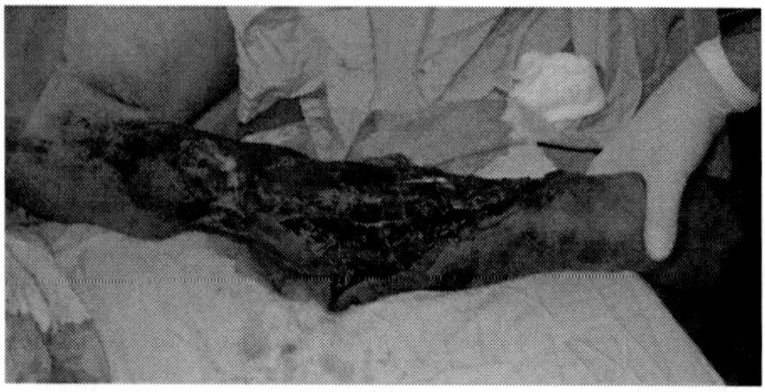

(a)

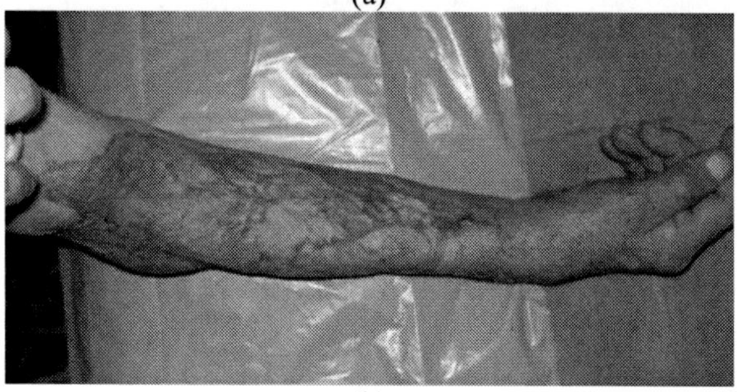

(b)

Figure 2. A. Mangled upper extremity. B. After skin graft.

Sequelae Following Untreated Compartment Syndrome in the Upper Extremity

The effect of hypoxia in the ischemic phase of acute compartment syndrome is the development of an acidic environment. In this circumstances, myoglobin is released from the ischemic muscle. Acute renal failure and tubular necrosis are the results of myoglobin precipitation in the nephron [37].

Locally, untreated compartment syndrome in the upper extremity could result in Volkmann's contracture. This is an ischemic muscle contracture due to injury leading to functional loss of the upper limb. The pathophysiology of Volkmann's contracture begins with hypertension in the venous part of the capillary beds, leading to obstruction at the capillary level. The arterial flow continues and causes increasing intracompartmental pressure. Volkmann's contracture develops more frequently in the volar compartment of the forearm due to non-compliant surrounding structures [38].

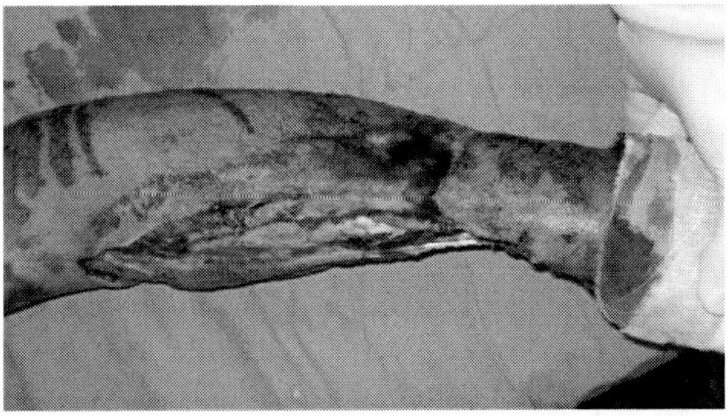

(a)

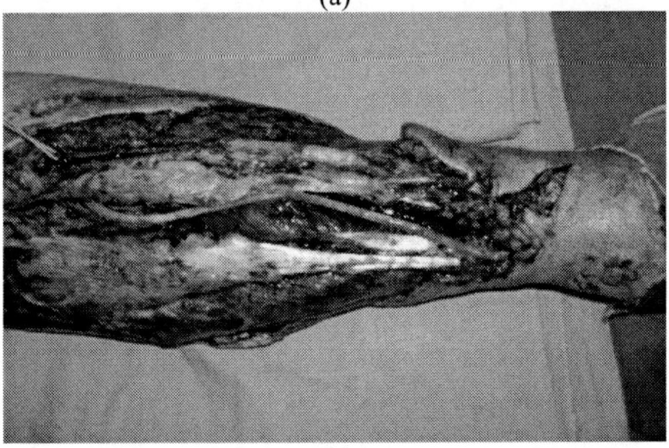

(b)

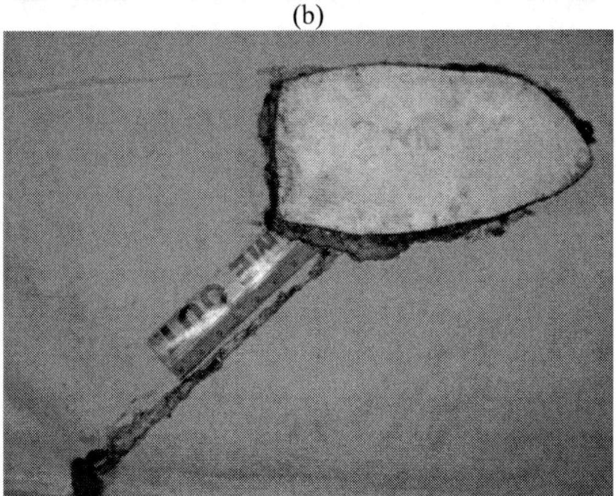

(c)

Figure 3. (Continued).

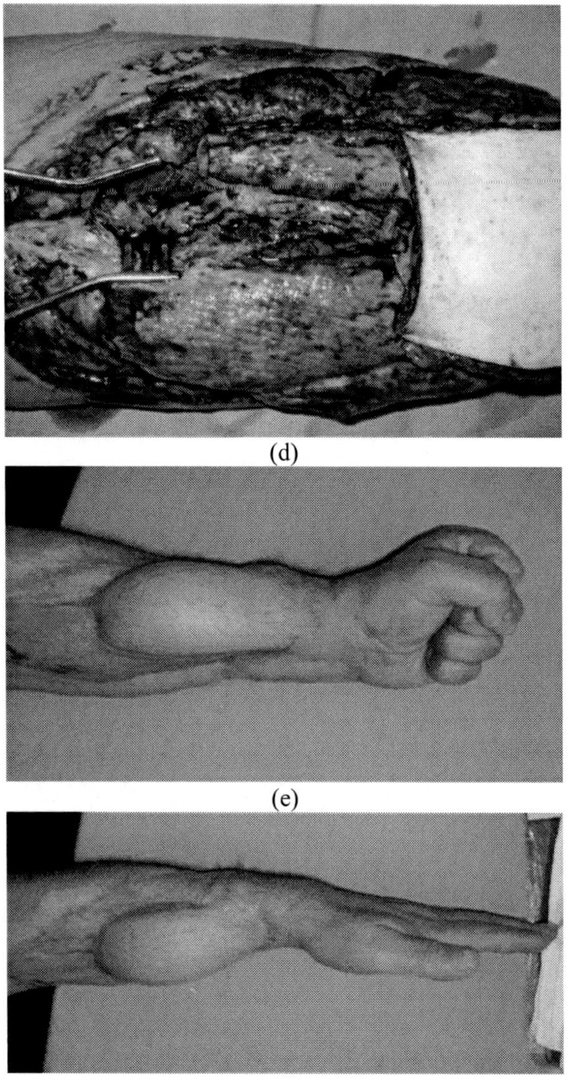

(d)

(e)

(f)

Figure 3. A. Working accident associated with soft tissue loss, radius fracture radial artery and ulnar artery injury, median nerve injury and flexor tendons injury. B. After debridement, tendon repair, nerve repair and revascularization using vein graft. C. Anteromedial thigh flap was harvested for soft tissue coverage. D. Anastomoses of the flap. E. One year later – full flexion. F. Full tendon extension.

Clinically, upper limb deformity due to ischemic contracture is characterized by elbow flexion, forearm pronation, wrist angulation, interphalangeal joint flexion and metacarpophalangeal joint extension.

Nonoperative management with rehabilitation therapy for increasing motion and strength is indicated in mild contracture. In some cases, operative treatment is necessary: devitalized muscle excision and tendon lengthening [39].

In cases of moderate or severe ischemic contracture, the surgical management steps are:

1) Nerve decompression: median and ulnar [40]
2) Tendon lengthening by direct method or by free-tissue transfer to restore lost function [41]
3) Free muscle transfers for rehabilitation of upper extremity function [42]

References

[1] Gourgiotis, S; Villias, C; Germanos, S; Foukas, A; Ridolfini, MP. Acute limb compartment syndrome: a review. *J. Surg. Educ.*, 64(3), 178-186 (2007).

[2] Mabvuure, NT; Malahias, M; Hindocha, S; Khan, W; Juma, A. Acute compartment syndrome of the limbs: current concepts and management. *Open Orthop. J.*, 6, 535-543, 2012.

[3] Allen, MJ; Stirling, AJ; Crawshaw, CV; Barnes, MR. MR. Intracompartmental pressure monitoring of leg injuries. An aid to management. *J. Bone Joint Surg. Br.*, 67(1), 53-57 (1985).

[4] Bumbasirevic, M; Stevanovic, M; Lesic, A; Atkinson, HD. Current management of the mangled upper extremity. *Int. Orthop.*, 36(11), 2189-2195 (2012).

[5] Prasarn, ML; Helfet, DL; Kloen, P. Management of the mangled extremity. *Strategies Trauma Limb Reconstr.*, 7(2), 57-66 (2012).

[6] Johansen, K; Daines, M; Howey, T; Helfet, D; Hansen, ST. ST Jr. Objective criteria accurately predict amputation following lower extremity trauma. *J. Trauma.*, 30(5), 568-573 (1990).

[7] Korompilias, AV; Beris, AE; Lykissas, MG; Vekris, MD; Kontogeorgakos, VA; Soucacos, PN. The mangled extremity and attempt for limb salvage. *J. Orthop. Surg. Res.*, 4, 4 (2009).

[8] Fagelman, MF; Epps, HR; Rang, M. Mangled extremity severity score in children. *J. Pediatr. Orthop.*, 22(2), 182-184 (2002).

[9] Fodor, L; Sobec, R; Sita-Alb, L; Fodor, M; Ciuce, C. C. Mangled lower extremity: can we trust the amputation scores? *Int. J. Burns Trauma.*, 2(1), 51-58 (2012).

[10] Owens, BD; Kragh Jr, JF; Wenke, JC; Macaitis, J; Wade, CE; Holcomb, JB. Combat wounds in operation Iraqi Freedom and operation Enduring Freedom. *J. Trauma.*, 64(2), 295-299 (2008).

[11] Peik, SM; Pollack, KM; Canham-Chervak, M; Hauret, KG; Baker, SP. Injuries to deployed U.S. Army soldiers involved in HMMWV crashes, 2002-2006. *Mil. Med.*, 177(8), 963-969 (2012).

[12] Dorlac, WC; DeBakey, ME; Holcomb, JB; Fagan, SP; Kwong, KL; Dorlac, GR; Schreiber, MA; Persse, DE; Moore, FA; Mattox, KL. Mortality from isolated civilian penetrating extremity injury. *J. Trauma.*, 59(1), 217-222 (2005).

[13] Franz, RW; Goodwin, RB; Hartman, JF; Wright, ML. Management of upper extremity arterial injuries at an urban level I trauma center. *Ann. Vasc. Surg.*, 23(1), 8-16 (2009).

[14] Kauvar, DS; Sarfati, MR; Kraiss, LW. National trauma databank analysis of mortality and limb loss in isolated lower extremity vascular trauma. *J. Vasc. Surg.*, 53(6), 1598-1603 (2011).

[15] Ball, CG; Rozycki, GS; Feliciano, DV. Upper extremity amputations after motor vehicle rollovers. *J. Trauma.*, 67(2), 410-412 (2009).

[16] Prichayudh, S; Verananvattna, A; Sriussadaporn, S; Sriussadaporn, S; Kritayakirana, K; Pak-art, R; Capin, A; Pereira, B; Tsunoyama, T. Pena. D. Management of upper extremity vascular injury: outcome related to the Mangled Extremity Severity Score. *World J. Surg.*, 33(4), 857-863 (2009).

[17] Burkhart, KJ; Mueller, LP; Prommersberger, K-J; Rommens, PM. Acute compartment syndrome of the upper extremity. *Eur. J. Trauma Emerg. Surg.*, 33, 584-588 (2007).

[18] Standring, S. *Gray's Anatomy,* 40th edition. Elsevier (2008).

[19] DiFelice, Jr A; Seiler, 3rd JG; Whitesides, Jr TE. The compartments of the hand: an anatomic study. *J. Hand Surg. Am.*, 23(4), 682-686 (1998).

[20] Ling, MZ; Kumar, VP. Myofascial compartments of the hand in relation to compartment syndrome: a cadaveric study. *Plast. Reconstr. Surg.*, 123(2), 613-616 (2009).

[21] Dente, CJ; Feliciano, DV; Rozycki, GS; Cava, RA; Ingram, WL; Salomone, JP; Nicholas, JM; Kanakasundaram, D; Ansley, JP. A review

of upper extremity fasciotomies in a level I trauma center. *Am. Surg.*, 70(12), 1088-1093 (2004).

[22] Ciclamini, D; Panero, B; Titolo, P; Tos, P; Battiston, B. Particularities of hand and wrist complex injuries in polytrauma management. *Injury.*, 45(2), 448-451 (2014).

[23] Kanj, WW; Gunderson, MA; Carrigan, RB; Sankar, WN. Acute compartment syndrome of the upper extremity in children: diagnosis, management, and outcomes. *J. Child. Orthop.*, 7(3), 225-233 (2013).

[24] Whitesides, Jr TE; Haney, TC; Harada, H; Holmes, HE; Morimoto, K. A simple method for tissue pressure determination. *Arch. Surg.*, 110(11), 1311-1313 (1975).

[25] Whitesides, TE; Heckman, MM. Acute compartment syndrome: Update on diagnosis and treatment. *J. Am. Acad. Orthop. Surg.*, 4(4), 209-218 (1996).

[26] Gulgonen, A; Ozer, K. Compartment syndrome, in *Greens's Operative Hand Surgery,* 6th edition. Elsevier. 1929-1948 (2011).

[27] Nelson, JA. Compartment pressure measurements have poor specificity for compartment syndrome in the traumatized limb. *J. Emerg. Med.*, 44(5), 1039-1044 (2013).

[28] Boody, AR; Wongworawat, MD. Accuracy in the measurement of compartment pressures: a comparison of three commonly used devices. *J. Bone Joint Surg.*, 87(11), 2415-2422 (2005).

[29] Wall, CJ; Lynch, J; Harris, IA; Richardson, MD; Brand, C; Lowe, AJ; Sugrue, M; Liverpool (Sydney) and Royal Melbourne Hospitals. Clinical practice guidelines for the management of acute limb compartment syndrome following trauma. *ANZ J. Surg.*, 80(3), 151-156 (2010).

[30] Garfin, SR; Mubarak, SJ; Evans, KL; Hargens, AR; Akeson, WH. Quantification of intracompartmental pressure and volume under plaster casts. *J. Bone Joint Surg. Am.*, 63(3), 449-453 (1981).

[31] Klenerman, L. The evolution of the compartment syndrome since 1948 as recorded in the JBJS (B). *J. Bone Joint Surg. Br.*, 89(10), 1280-1282 (2007).

[32] Kostler, W; Strohm, PC; Sudkamp, NP. Acute compartment syndrome of the limb. *Injury.*, 35(12), 1221-1227 (2004).

[33] Mubarak, SJ; Hargens, AR. Acute compartment syndromes. *Surg. Clin. North Am.*, 63(3), 539-565 (1983).

[34] Ouellette, EA; Kelly, R. Compartment syndromes of the hand. *J. Bone Joint Surg. Am.*, 78(10), 1515-1522 (1996).

[35] Ojike, NI; Roberts, CS; Giannoudis, PV. Compartment syndrome of the thigh: a systematic review. *Injury.*, 41(2), 133-136 (2010).

[36] Sayar, U; Ozer, T; Mataraci, I. Forearm compartment syndrome caused by reperfusion injury. *Case Rep. Vasc. Med.*, 2014, 931410 (2014).

[37] Prasarn, ML; Ouellette, EA. Acute compartment syndrome of the upper extremity. *J. Am. Acad. Orthop. Surg.*, 19(1), 49-58 (2011).

[38] Reigstad, A; Hellum, C. Volkmann's ischaemic contracture of the forearm. *Injury.*, 12(2), 148-150 (1980).

[39] Botte, MJ; Keenan, MA; Gelberman, RH. Volkmann's ischemic contracture of the upper extremity. *Hand Clin.*, 14(3), 483-497 (1998).

[40] Urban, J. [Median nerve decompression in ischemic contracture of the forearm]. *Chir. Narzadow Ruchu. Ortop. Pol.*, 64(6), 609-613 (1999).

[41] Ultee, J; Hovius, SE. Functional results after treatment of Volkmann's ischemic contracture: a long-term followup study. *Clin. Orthop. Relat. Res.* (431), 42-49 (2005).

[42] Fischer, JP;. Elliott, RM; Kozin, SH; Levin, LS. Free function muscle transfers for upper extremity reconstruction: a review of indications, techniques, and outcomes. *J. Hand Surg. Am.*, 38(12), 2485-2490 (2013).

In: Compartment Syndrome
Editor: Anna P. Henderson

ISBN: 978-1-63482-831-4

Chapter 5

Lower Limb Compartment Syndrome Associated with Vascular Injuries

***Marius Fodor*[1,*]*, Olimpiu Bota*[2] *and Lucian Fodor*[2]**
[1]Department of General Surgery, Emergency District Hospital, Cluj-Napoca, Romania
[2]Department of Plastic and Reconstructive Surgery, Emergency District Hospital, Cluj- Napoca, Romania

Abstract

Lower limb vascular injuries are often present in severe trauma. Frequently, the vascular lesions are associated with lower limb bone fractures, muscle contusion or rupture, burns and external limb compression. Among the most common causes are acute injuries by sharp objects, car accidents and fractures. Vein injuries are less often present but are possible in severe compartment syndrome. All these can lead to acute compartment syndrome due to intramuscular hematomas and soft tissue edema. Compartment syndrome of the lower limb is a clinical entity resulting from increased pressure in a non-expansile tissue space and is associated with significant morbidity and mortality. The diagnosis of compartment syndrome combined with vascular trauma in the lower

[*] Corresponding author: Email: Marius Fodor – drfodor@yahoo.com.

limb is mostly clinical and by measurements of the compartment pressure. Diagnosis can be delayed in unconscious patients. It is of paramount importance to identify this problem and treat it as soon as possible. There are important predictor factors for fasciotomy: multi-system trauma, open fractures and knee dislocation associated with vascular injury. Herein we detail the step-by-step guide for identifying compartment syndrome in conscious and unconscious patients with lower limb vascular injuries and modalities of treatment.

Compartment Syndrome (CS) is a constellation of clinical signs and symptoms which occur when the pressure inside a fascial compartment exceeds that of the tissue perfusion pressure, leading to loss of function and, in severe cases, loss of limb, and is potentially life-threatening. The pathophysiology of CS includes a breakdown of the local homeostasis with decreased capillary perfusion and increased tissue pressure, leading to ischemia and tissue necrosis [1] (Figure 1). CS can be caused by conditions which increase the compartment volume, the most frequent being fractures, followed by soft tissue injuries, revascularization and fluid infusions, or by conditions which reduce the compartment volume, such as burns, dressings and casts [1].

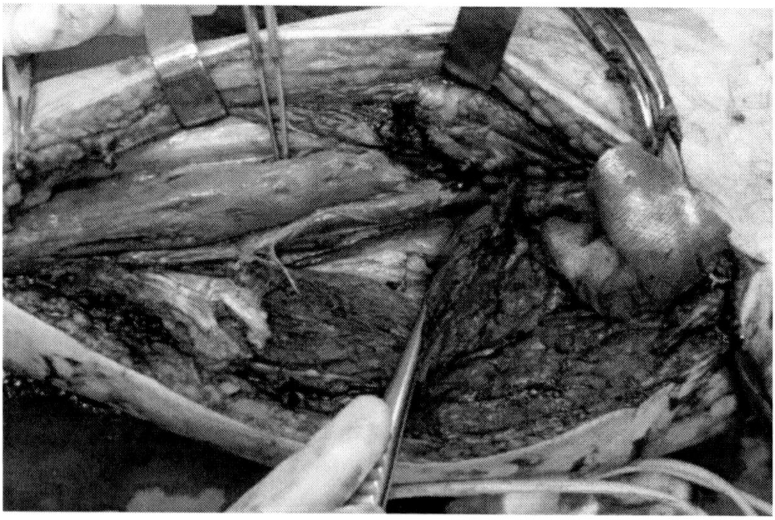

Figure 1. Calf trauma – late presentation. Four days after compartment syndrome with partial muscle necrosis; the different colour (grey) of the necrotic muscle can be seen in the upper part.

Important Lower Limb Anatomy

The Gluteal Region

The complex bony structure of the pelvis serves to host the abdominal organs during upright ambulation, and the bony prominences of the pelvis serve as muscle attachments. The fascial system of the gluteal region and the lower extremity contain a superficial fascial and a deep fascial layer. The superficial system is located within the subcutaneous fat, usually as a dividing layer where superficial veins and nerves traverse to reach the overlying skin. The deep fascial layer is thicker and frequently can be seen as a dual-layered fibrous band.

The superficial fascia of the gluteal region continues the lower back fascia into the proximal thigh. The deep fascia covering the gluteal muscles forms the thick, strong, gluteal aponeurosis which is attached to the lateral border of the iliac crest superiorly, and splits anteriorly to enclose the tensor fasciae latae and posteriorly to enclose the gluteus maximus. The gluteus maximus muscle acts as a hip extensor. Its innervation comes from the inferior gluteal nerve and the blood supply is provided mainly by the inferior gluteal artery, as well as the superior gluteal vessels and the first perforator of the profunda femoris. The gluteus medius abducts the hip and medially rotates the femur and is vascularized by the inferior gluteal artery and innervated by the superior gluteal nerve. The gluteus minimus abducts the hip and is vascularized by the superior gluteal artery and innervated by the superior gluteal nerve. Other smaller muscles, which include the piriformis, superior and inferior gemellus, quadratus femoris, obturator internus, and obturator externus, collectively rotate the hip externally.

The gluteal muscles are supplied by the gluteal vessels. The superior gluteal artery arises as the last branch of the posterior trunk of the internal iliac artery and courses through the greater sciatic foramen above the piriformis muscle, dividing into two branches. Both branches supply the muscles and the skin in this area and finally connect with branches from the lateral circumflex femoral artery. The inferior gluteal artery arises from the anterior part of the internal iliac artery and passes through the greater sciatic foramen inferior to the piriformis muscle, to supply the gluteus maximus muscle and the overlying skin.

The innervation of the gluteal region and upper thigh is supplied by the posterior cutaneous nerve of the thigh and the gluteal nerves. The first one arises from S1 to S3 and innervates the skin of the buttocks and the posterior thigh. The superior gluteal nerve runs with the superior gluteal artery and divides into two branches which run with the respective branches of the superior gluteal artery and innervates the gluteus medius and minimus muscles as well as the tensor fascia latae. The inferior gluteal nerve runs with the inferior gluteal artery and innervates the gluteus maximus muscle [1, 2].

The Thigh

The thigh has the function of sustaining the trunk and positioning the knee. The fascial system of the thigh is composed from superficial and deep fascia. The superficial fascia is relatively thin but thickens in the inguinal region. It merges with the deep fascia at the inguinal ligament. The deep fascia is a thick, well-vascularized, fibrous tissue which encompasses the whole thigh muscles. It inserts on the pelvic bones and inguinal ligament and gives away septa which pass to the bone and form three osteofascial compartments, which provide an additional insertion to the muscles and form functional units which enhance muscle efficiency. The medial and lateral intermuscular septa separate the anterior and posterior compartments, which contain the knee extensor and knee flexor muscles. The medial compartment has no defined intermuscular septa and contains the adductor muscles of the thigh.

Beneath the inguinal ligament lies the fossa ovalis, which is an opening in both fascia, allowing the great saphenous vein, superficial branches of the femoral artery and the lymphatics to pass through. The fossa ovalis is covered with a membranous layer of the superficial fascia, called the cribriform fascia. The deep fascia becomes very thick on the lateral aspect of the thigh and is called the iliotibial tract. Its role is to maintain knee extension.

The iliopsoas muscle originates from the lumbar vertebral column and inserts on the femur, flexing the thigh. The anterior thigh compartment contains the sartorius, articularis genu and quadriceps muscles, represented by the rectus femoris, vastus lateralis, intermedius and medialis. They are primary knee extensors, except for the sartorius and rectus femoris which originate on the pelvis and also flex the thigh.

The posterior compartment of the thigh contains three muscles, biceps femoris laterally and semitendinous and semimembranous medially. The long head of the first one extends the hip and all three muscles flex the knee. The adductor compartment is positioned medially and contains the adductor magnus, brevis, longus and the gracilis and pectineus muscles. On the lateral side of the thigh, not included in one of the three compartments, lies the tensor fascia lata muscle. Its role is to stabilize the knee through the iliotibial tract.

The main blood supply for the thigh is represented by the femoral artery. It continues the iliac external iliac artery while crossing under the inguinal ligament and passes to the femoral canal, where it lies next to the femoral vein in the femoral sheath which represents the continuation of the transversalis and the femoral fasciae. In this area, the femoral vessels are found in the so-called femoral triangle, which is marked laterally by the sartorius muscle, medially by the adductor longus muscle and superiorly by the inguinal ligament. They lie on the pectineus and iliopsoas muscles. In this space, 4cm inferior to the inguinal ligament, they divide into two branches, the deep and the superficial femoral arteries. After they cross beneath the sartorius muscle, the superficial femoral vessels pass into the femoral (Hunter's) canal, which is a fibromuscular canal formed laterally by the vastus medialis, medially by the adductor lungus and magnus and anterior by the sartorius.

The deep femoral artery (profunda fermoris) represents the main vascular supply to the thigh. It originates from the common femoral artery. The profunda femoris passes between the vastus medialis and the adductor magnus muscles. After the origin, it branches to the medial and lateral circumflex arteries. It also gives rise to four perforating branches which pass through the adductor magnus muscle and vascularize the adductor and posterior compartments.

Motor innervation is realized by three nerves, each one supplying one compartment: the femoral nerve for the anterior compartment, the obturator nerve for the adductor compartment, and the sciatic nerve for the posterior compartment. The femoral nerves originates from L2-L4, passes beneath the inguinal canal lateral to the femoral vessels and divides into posterior and anterior branches. It terminates with the saphenous nerve.

The obturator nerve also originates from L2-L4,and passes through the obturator foramen. It divides into two branches. The posterior branch innervates the adductor magnus and part of the knee joint. The anterior branch innervates the adductor longus, brevis, gracilis and the hip joint.

The sciatic nerve arises from L4-S3, passes through the sciatic foramen beneath the piriformis muscle and divides into the tibial and common peroneal nerves. The first nerve innervates all the posterior compartment muscles, except for the short head of the biceps muscle, which is innervated by the latter.

The lateral cutaneous nerve of the thigh arises from the L2-L3, travels underneath or through the inguinal ligament and divides into two branches which innervate the anterolateral side of the thigh. The posterior femoral cutaneous nerve originates from S1-S3. It passes through the greater sciatic foramen and innervates the inferior gluteal region and the posterior thigh. The terminal branches and contributes to the sural nerve.

The femoral nerve forms from its anterior division, the intermediate cutaneous and medial cutaneous nerves of the thigh, which innervate the anteromedial side of the thigh. The anterior division of the oburator nerve innervates the inferomedial portion of the thigh [3-5].

The Calf

The bone structure of the calf is formed by the tibia and fibula. The patella is the largest sesamoid bone in the body and is part of the knee joint. This is formed by two joints, the tibiofemoral and the patellofemural joints. Although most weight-bearing is done by the tibia, the tibiofibular joint takes about one-sixth of the axial load of the leg.

The calf has also a superficial and a deep fascial system. The superficial fascia contains the greater and lesser saphenous veins as well as the saphenous and sural nerves. The deep fascia encompasses the whole leg and has different thicknesses, with the posterior part being the thinner and more pliable part. Proximally it is adherent to the tibial tuberosity, fibular head and the patellar tendon. Posteriorly it is thicker and covers the popliteal fossa, being called here the popliteal fascia. In this area the lesser saphenous vein and the sural nerve pass from the subcutaneous tissue through the fascia towards the popliteal space.

The tibiofibular interosseus membrane is an oblique fibrous structure between the two bones. It separates the anterior and posterior muscle compartments and serves as a muscle insertion on both sides. In the superior part it forms the oval aperture which allows the anterior tibial vessels to pass into the anterior compartment. The inferior part also forms a passage for the perforating branches from the distal peroneal artery.

The deep fascia sends several septa to the bones which divide the leg into four compartments. The anterior compartment is bounded medially by the tibia, posteriorly by the interosseous membrane and laterally by the anterior intermuscular septum, which separates it from the lateral compartment. The lateral compartment lies on the fibula and is separated posteriorly by the posterior intermuscular septum from the posterior compartment. The posterior compartment is divided by the transverse intermuscular septum into a superficial compartment and a deep posterior compartment, which lies posterior to the interosseous membrane.

The anterior compartment comprises the following muscles: tibialis anterior, extensor digitorum longus, extensor hallucis longus and peroneus tertius. Their action is to dorsiflex the ankle, foot and toes. The lateral compartment contains the peroneus longus and brevis, with the former being more superficial than the latter. Both muscles act to evert and plantar flex the foot. The posterior superficial compartment contains the medial and lateral gastrocnemius, soleus and plantaris muscles, which all plantar flex the ankle and, except for the soleus, flex the knee.

The deep posterior compartment contains the following muscles: popliteus, flexor digitorum longus, flexor hallucis longus and tibialis posterior. They lie beneath the transverse fascia. The flexor digitorum and hallucis longus have interconnected tendons and act as plantar flexors of the foot and toes. The tibialis posterior lies on the interosseous membrane and plantar flexes the ankle and foot.

The vascularity of the leg emerges from the popliteal artery, which represents the continuation of the superficial femoral artery after exiting the adductor canal. Around the knee the artery has multiple genicular branches, which anastomose and form a plexus with the recurrent branches from the tibial and peroneal arteries. Before exiting the popliteal space, the popliteal artery gives off its first terminal branch, the anterior tibial artery which passes through the oval foramen into the anterior compartment, where it vascularizes all the muscles.

After passing beneath the popliteus muscle, the popliteal artery branches into the posterior tibial and peroneal arteries, which then course in the deep posterior compartment, with the peroneal artery lying close to the fibula. The peroneal artery terminates through a perforating branch which passes at the distal level of the interosseous membrane anteriorly and anastomoses with the anterior tibial artery. The posterior tibial artery becomes more superficial in the lower third of the calf, passing then behind the medial malleolus where it gives its terminal braches: the medial and lateral plantar arteries. The muscles of the posterior compartments are vascularized by the peroneal and tibial arteries as well as from the two sural arteries, branches of the popliteal artery. The lateral compartment is vascularized through septal branches from the anterior tibial and peroneal arteries.

Most of the innervation of the calf is derived from the sciatic nerve. It bifurcates into two main branches at different levels of the thigh or popliteal space: the posterior tibial and the common peroneal nerves. The former runs through the deep posterior compartment together with the posterior tibial artery and innervates the muscles in both posterior compartments. At the level of the malleolus it bifurcates into the medial and lateral plantar nerves, which innervate the foot muscles and the sole.

The common peroneal nerve passes from the popliteal fossa around the fibular neck, underneath the long peroneal muscle, into the anterior compartment. At this level it bifurcates into the superficial peroneal nerve and the deep peroneal nerve. The first one travels between the peroneus muscles, which it innervates and then becomes superficial, pierces the fascia and innervates the lower lateral leg and the foot dorsum. The deep peroneal nerve travels in front of the interosseous membrane and innervates all the muscles in the anterior compartment. At the level of the ankle it is found next to the tibial artery and then gives articular branches and a sensitive branch to the first interdigital space.

The saphenous nerve, terminal branch of the femoral nerve, innervates the medial leg. The medial sural nerve, branching from the tibial nerve, supplies the medial posterior leg and the lateral sural nerve supplies the lateral posterior leg. The proper sural nerve is constituted from several communicating branches, which coalesce and run down the posterior face of the leg, innervating the distal posterior third of the leg and the lateral side of the foot [3-5].

The Ankle and Foot

The foot and ankle have seven tarsal bones – talus, calcaneus, cuboid, navicular and medial, intermediate and lateral cuneiforms. The ankle is composed of two joints, one between the distal surfaces of the tibia and fibula and the superior face of the talus and the subtalar joint, and one between the inferior surface of the talus and the calcaneus.

At the level of the ankle, the fascial system forms three retinacula, whose role is to group the tendons and prevent bowstringing. On the dorsal side there is the extensor retinaculum, which has two parts. The superior extensor retinaculum retains the extensor digitorum and hallucis longus, the tibialis anterior and peroneus tertius tendons. The anterior tibial artery and the deep peroneal nerve pass beneath it. The inferior part is Y-shaped, with its origin on the lateral side of calcaneus. The medial part bifurcates. The superior part retains the extensor hallucis longus and tibialis anterior tendons and the inferior part the peroneus tertius, the extensor digitorum longus, the extensor hallucis longus tendons, the anterior tibial vessels and the deep peroneal nerve.

The flexor retinaculum spreads from the medial malleolus towards the calcaneus and plantar aponeurosis. It retains the flexor digitorum longus, flexor hallucis longus and tibialis posterior tendons, the posterior tibial vessels and the tibial nerve. The tendons are usually placed anteriorly and the neurovascular bundle posteriorly. The peroneal retinaculum retains the long and short peroneal tendons.

After forming the retinacula, the fascial system encompasses the foot, giving multiple extensions to the tarsal and metatarsal bones and to the skin, to form multiple functional compartments. In the foot, the fascia becomes very thick and forms the plantar fascia, which constrains the underlying structures and provides stable support for the overlying glabrous skin.

There are three plantar compartments and one interosseous compartment. The medial plantar compartment contains the abductor hallucis and flexor hallucis muscle. The central compartment contains the flexor digitorum brevis, quadratus plantae and the adductor hallucis muscles. The lateral plantar compartment contains the abductor digiti minimi and the flexor digiti minimi. The multiple divisions of the plantar arteries and nerves are contained within these compartments. The interosseous compartment contains the intrinsic muscles between the first and fifth metatarsals.

The foot contains extrinsic muscles which originate in the leg and intrinsic muscles, which act primarily on the toes and secondarily stabilize the osteocartilaginous architecture of the foot. The plantar muscles are organized in multiple layers. The first layer, situated directly under the plantar aponeurosis, contains the abductor hallucis, flexor digitorum brevis and adductor digiti minimi.

Underneath this layer run the tendons of the flexor digitorum and hallucis longus, as well as the medial and lateral plantar arteries and nerves, which divide here into their terminal branches. The second muscular layer contains the quadratus plantae muscle, which originates from the calcaneus and inserts on the flexor digitorum longus tendons, aiding with the plantar flexion and lumbrical muscles, which originate on the medial side of the extensor digitorum longus and insert on the extensor system.

The third layer contains the flexor hallucis brevis, the adductor hallucis and the flexor digiti minimi brevis muscles. The fourth layer contains the three plantar interossei, which adduct the toes and the four dorsal interossei, which abduct the toes. The dorsum of the foot contains the extensor digitorum and hallucis brevis.

The vascularization of the foot is provided by the dorsalis pedis, tibialis posterior arteries, and the terminal branches of the peroneal artery.

The dorsalis pedis continues the anterior tibial artery. It runs beneath the retinaculum extensorum and is then positioned on the dorsum of the foot between the extensor hallucis and digitorum longus tendons. Distally it gives off a perforating branch which passes between the first and second metatarsals and anastomoses with the lateral plantar artery, to form the plantar arch. It also gives off the first dorsal intermetatarsal artery and supplies the proximal dorsum of the foot.

The posterior tibial artery bifurcates at the level the ankle into the medial and lateral plantar arteries. The medial plantar artery has a smaller caliber and contributes to the blood supply of the first toes. The lateral plantar artery is the dominant blood supply to the foot and forms, together with the perforating branch from the dorsalis pedis, the plantar arch which gives off metatarsal branches which vascularize the toes.

The peroneal artery's terminal branches anastomose with the lateral malleolar and calcaneal branches from the tibial artery to supply the ankle region. When the other two arteries of the foot are deficient, the peroneal artery may augment its flow to supply the foot with blood.

The motor innervation of the foot is supplied by the deep peroneal nerve, which innervates the extensor digitorum and hallucis brevis. The medial plantar nerve innervates the abductor hallucis, flexor hallucis and digitorum brevis and the first lumbrical muscles, as well as the skin from the first to the third toes.

The lateral plantar nerve innervates the interossei muscles, second through fourth lumbricals, adductor hallucis, quadratus plantae, abductor digiti minimi, flexor digiti minimi brevis, and the skin for the fourth and fifth toes.

The cutaneous innervation of the dorsum and sides of the foot is supplied by the superficial and deep peroneal, saphenous and sural nerves, as discussed in the calf section.

The sole of the foot is supplied by the posterior tibial nerve through the medial calcaneal, medial plantar and lateral plantar nerves. Additionally, the proximal lateral edge of the foot sole is supplied by the lateral calcaneal nerve, a branch of the sural nerve, and the medial proximal edge of the foot sole is supplied by the saphenous nerve [3-5].

Causes of Vascular Injuries

A. Primary

The vascular injuries of the lower extremity may be produced directly, causing a primary lesion of the vessels. The cause in these cases may be either a penetrating (56-66%) or a blunt (34-44%) trauma [1, 2]. The most frequently encountered mechanism for penetrating trauma is gunshot wounds, followed by stab wounds. Iatrogenic injuries are a rare cause of vascular trauma.

Most studies indicate the superficial femoral artery as most frequently involved in vascular injuries of the lower extremity, followed by the tibial, popliteal, common femoral and deep femoral arteries. In about 19% of cases, more than one artery is injured [4,6].

According to the type of arterial injury, the mechanism may depend on the frequency occlusion, transection, laceration or dissection [1,2]. Associated lesions may include vein injury in 45% of cases, nerve injury in 16.4%, and bone fracture in 31.4% [1].

B. Secondary

Another cause of vascular injuries of the lower extremity is a secondary lesion of the vessels through a fractured bone. In a study on 136 patients, Topal et al., [7] found the incidence of associated fractures to be 31.4%, 24% being below-knee fractures, of which 41% were two bone fractures.

C. Late

In some cases, a primary incomplete arterial lesion with blood leakage into the adventia leads to the formation of a pseudaneurysm. This may rupture secondarily, leading to limb ischemia and CS. This phenomenon may also happen iatrogenically, after vascular injuries or dehiscent vascular sutures [2].

Clinical Features of Compartment Syndrome after Vascular Injuries of Lower Extremity

Acute compartment syndrome (ACS) can be present in all compartments of the lower limb. The anterior compartment of the calf is the most affected and visible. The diagnosis of ACS at onset is mainly clinically but this is not enough for an accurate early diagnosis. The main symptom during development of ACS is pain. The pain is described as out of proportion to the injury, increasing in intensity in time and resistant to common analgesics. Also, paresthesia, paresis and palpable tenseness are associated with the pain during development of ACS. Significant increased pain during tendon flexion/extension can be a sign of ACS.

In children and adults who have a modified level of consciousness, pain is not useful as a diagnostic tool for ACS. In this situation, direct measurement of intracompartmental pressure is important for a positive diagnosis [2]. Lack of a pulse and slow capillary refill are noted late in ACS and are associated with vascular trauma.

Usually, the diagnosis of ACS implies a high index of suspicion and requires a repeated clinical evaluation, due to gradually increasing intracompartmental pressure which determines, in time, neuromuscular hypoxia. Because of this evolution, it is mandatory to monitor intracompartmental pressure in the first 48 hours after bone fracture, when a high suspicion of compartment syndrome is raised.

Signs and symptoms of ACS are correlated with intracompartmental pressure (ICP). Normal ICP in the resting position is 0-8 mmHg. Local blood perfusion decreases when ICP increases. When ICP is above the capillary pressure (20-30 mmHg), the signs of ischemia are present. When the compartmental fascial membrane is maximally stretched at 30-33mmHg, ICP pressure and the compliance of the compartment is compromised. In this situation, most surgeons recommend fasciotomy [8].

ACS in the thigh is less reported than in the distal lower extremity, because a large volume of liquid is necessary to increase the ICP. The main causes of thigh ACS are massive hemorrhage and edema of the soft tissues [9]. Massive hemorrhage is caused by arterial injury, which determines rapid elevation of ICP with capillary compression leading to neuromuscular injury [10]. It is mandatory to treat the arterial lesion at the same time as the fasciotomy for compartment syndrome. A special situation concerning lower

limb ACS is related to a resuscitative maneuver in a patient with multiple trauma (head, thorax or abdominal trauma). Identification of lower extremity ACS in the unconscious patient is a challenge and needs repeated clinical and ICP examinations [11].

Differential Diagnosis of Compartment Syndrome Associated with Vascular Injuries

The differential diagnosis of ACS associated with vascular injuries should be made with:

1) Factors that increase compartment volume:
   Bone fracture, soft tissue trauma, crush syndrome, edema due to arterial revascularization, extensive muscle exercise, fluid infusion, vascular puncture, ruptured cyst, hypertrophy of ganglia, snake bite, viral myositis, leukemia, nephritic syndrome and deep vein thrombosis
2) Factors that reduce compartment volume:
   Surgery for muscle hernia, casts, burns, circumferential dressings
3) Associated diseases
   Diabetes mellitus, coagulation disorders, hypothyroidism [2, 12]

Bone fractures, regardless of the comminution, can be associated with increased ICP after surgical treatment (reduction of fracture, reaming or insertion of nail). The fascial tearing associated with a fracture is not enough to prevent ACS. Fracture fixation narrows the surrounding tissue, leading to a reduction of the compartmental volume and to an increase of the inside pressure. This aspect is well-known as the "finger-trap phenomenon" [13].

Application of a long leg cast increases the ICP. Soft-tissue edema and high elevation decreases the arteriovenous pressure gradient and, thus, the tissue becomes less tolerant of intracompartmental pressure. These aspects can explain the occurrence of ACS after surgery in the lithotomy or hemilithotomy positions [14].

In cases of deep vein thrombosis, erythema and collateral superficial veins can be noted, and ultrasound reveals thrombus in the posterior, anterior or peroneal veins.

Stress fracture is correlated with significant tenderness at the fracture site and x-ray shows bone discontinuity.

Acute ischemia of the lower extremity is associated with claudication and the absence of peripheral pulses. The Duplex ultrasound may present a peak systolic velocity ratio over 2 and a decreased pulsatility index between the proximal and distal leg segments.

Chronic venous insufficiency presents as varicose veins, and Duplex ultrasound demonstrates ostial valve closure time over 0.5 seconds (reflux).

Muscle tear is associated with tenderness and local ecchymosis. Ultrasound reveals hyperechogenicity, interruption of fibers in perimysial striae or a rounded appearance of the muscle stump. In all these situations, the ICP is normal. The differential diagnosis of compartmental syndrome in the lower extremity associated with vascular injury is very important for avoiding amputation [4, 15].

Treatment of Compartment Syndrome in the Lower Extremity

The main treatment of ACS in the lower extremity with vascular injury has two stages:

1) Reconstruction of injured vessels: direct suture, graft interposition or bypass
2) Extensive fasciotomy for muscle and nerve decompression
3) In the presence of severe crush syndrome, dialysis or plasma exchange should be taken into consideration [10, 11].

Trauma of the lower limb associated with hypotension and decreasing levels of hematocrit and hemoglobin is suspicious for an arterial lesion at the trauma site. This implies emergency treatment. Preoperative arteriography is useful for locating the arterial lesion and type of bone fracture.

The objective of fasciotomy is to relieve the increased pressure, thereby improving muscle perfusion and debriding necrotic tissue. Fasciotomy involves all compartments of the lower leg (Figure 2). The main types of fasciotomy are performed with single or double incisions. Some authors associate fasciotomy with partial fibular excision [16, 17]. The double incision technique implies no need to remove the bone and has less risk of trauma to neurovascular structures. It also makes good decompression of the posterior compartment. An 8cm skin incision reduced ICP from 48mm Hg to 25mmHg but, to adequately decompress all leg compartments, 12-20cm skin incisions are recommended [18].

A single incision is made on the fibular axis between 5cm from the fibular head to 5cm from the lateral malleous, followed by two fascial incisions, anteriorily and posteriorly, taking care of perforant vessels from skin flaps. Thus, all four compartments are fully decompressed. The dissection plane should be close to the fibula to avoid lesions of the peroneal artery and vein.

A double incision consists of anterolateral and posteromedial approaches. The anterolateral incision allows relaxing of the anterior compartment muscles, and the lateral compartment can be reached through the anterior intermuscular septum. The posteromedial incision made 2cm posterior to the tibial border decompresses the superficial and deep muscle compartments of the calf [8, 19]. A small incision and closed fasciotomy are rarely indicated in lower limb arterial injuries [20, 21]. When a soft tissue injury is associated with vascular injuries, using tension and forcing the skin wounds for closure is forbidden (Figures 3A, B, C). The moment of skin closure after fasciotomy depends on reducing the muscle swelling and surgically removing all necrotic tissue. Several methods of wound closure are reported:

1) Delayed primary wound closure
2) Split thickness skin graft is the most used technique
3) Skin stretching is done using skin staples or elastic cords which easily bring the skin margins together [22]
4) Vacuum-assisted wound closure can be useful for delayed primary wound closure or for applying a skin graft [23]

Complications and Sequelae Related to Compartment Syndrome in the Lower Extremity

There are a few reports concerning the long-term outcome after ACS in the lower extremity. Frink et al., [24] studied 26 patients with multiple trauma lesions of the lower leg who needed fasciotomy for ACS. After one year of follow-up, they found a decrease of isokinetic strength and work in the dorsal extensors and reduced power in the plantar flexors.

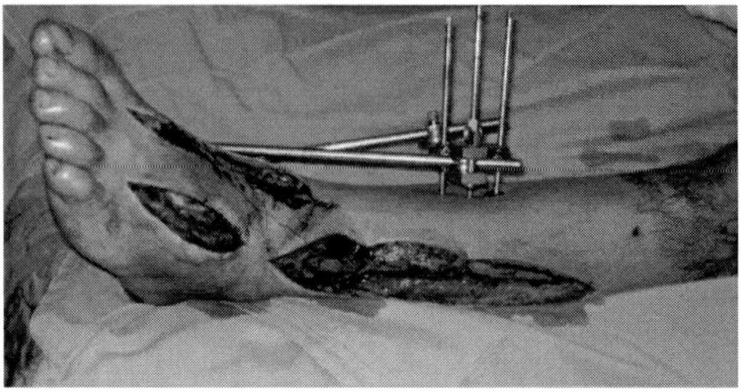

Figure 2. Calf and foot fasciotomies after vascular injuries. Fasciotomy of the medial part was also performed but cannot be seen in these views.

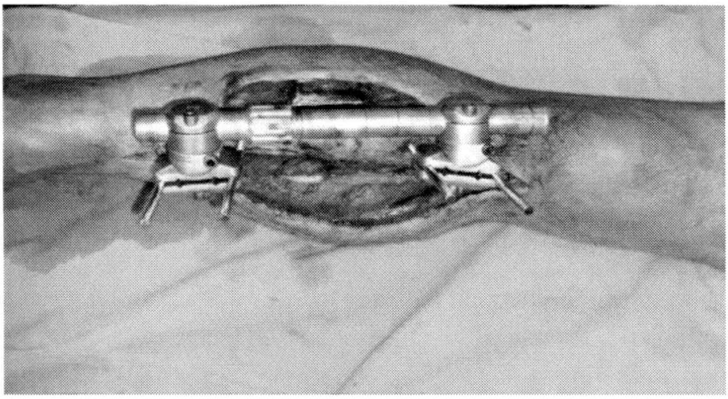

(a)

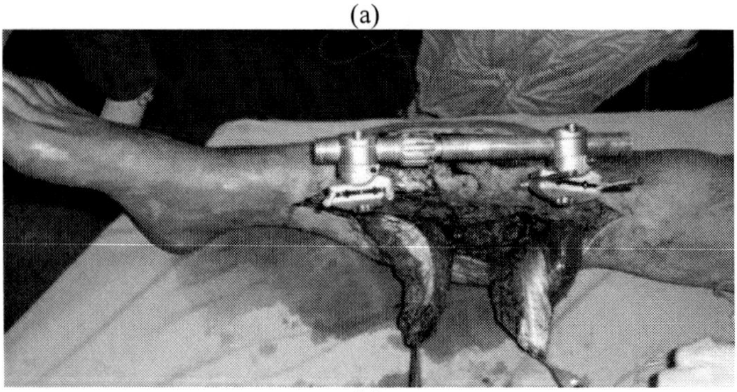

(b)

Figure 3. (Continued).

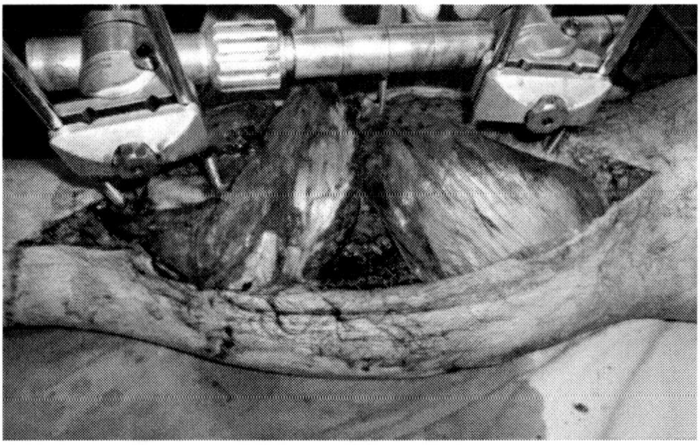

(c)

Figure 3. A - Complex calf trauma with tibial fracture and vascular injury. After revascularization and external bone fixation, there is a soft tissue defect. B - Local muscle flaps were preferred to cover exposed bone. Primary wound closure by placing force is forbidden. C - The exposed bone is complete covered.

Giannoudis et al., [25] studied the quality of life in patients with ACS of the lower extremity after trauma and used the EQ-5D (EuroQol) test after one year of follow-up. They noted that patients without skin grafts had fewer problems than patients with skin graft after fasciotomy for ACS. This study showed that ACS has a long-term impact on the patient's quality of life.

The main long-term sequelae after lower leg fasciotomy are dry and scaly skin with pruritus and neurologic manifestation (diminishing sensation and paresthesia) [26].

Frink et al., [24] studied 26 patients with fasciotomy and reported pain in the rest position (15.4%) and on exercise (26.9%).

The rate of infection after fasciotomy was reported to be as high as 38% [27].

Schepsis et al., [28] demonstrated that the anterior compartment of calf is more affected than the posterior compartment after fasciotomy.

Concerning foot sequelae after fasciotomy, discomfort on walking was noted and, in rare situations, foot contracture with claw toes was found.

The main long-term sequelae after fasciotomy of the lower extremity remains paresthesia and numbness [29].

When not recognized, ischemia and compartment syndrome can lead to amputation (Figures 4A, B).

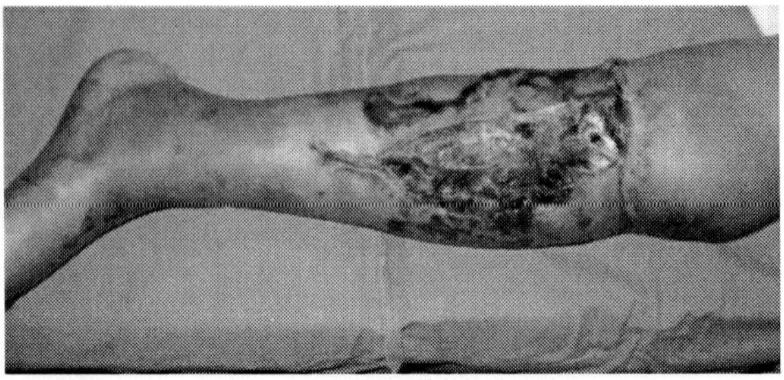

(a)

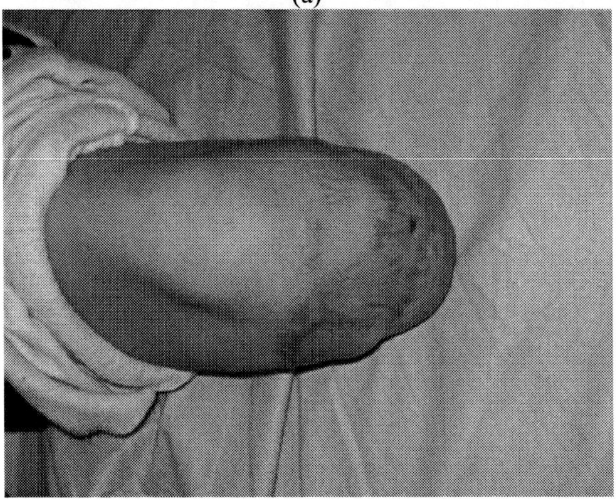

(b)

Figure 4. A - 30 hours after ischemia and compartment syndrome. Please note the typical foot color produced by ischemia. B - Below knee amputation was performed.

References

[1] Garner, M. R., Taylor, S. A., Gausden, E. & Lyden, J. P. (2014). Compartment syndrome: diagnosis, management& unique concerns in the twenty-first century. *HSS. J.*, *10*(2), 143-152.

[2] Shadgan, B., Menon, M., Sanders, D., Berry, G., Martin, Jr C., Duffy, P., Stephen, D. & O'Brien, P. J. (2010). Current thinking about acute compartment syndrome of the lower extremity. *Can. J. Surg.*, *53*(5), 329-334.

[3] Hansen, J. T. & Netter. F. H. (2010). *Netter's Clinical Anatomy*, 2nd edition. Saunders.

[4] Ginard, I. H. & Grant. M. K. (2013). Comprehensive lower extremity anatomy, in: P. C. Neligan and D. H. Song, editors. *Plastic Surgery*, 3rd edition, Volume 4, Elsevier Saunders Publishing.

[5] Gray, H. (2013). *Gray's Anatomy*, 15th edition. Guild of Master Craftsmen.

[6] Franz, R. W., Shah, K. J., Halaharvi, D., Franz, E. T., Hartman, J. F. & Wright, M. L. (2011). A 5-year review of management of lower extremity arterial injuries at an urban level I trauma center. *J. Vasc. Surg.*, *53*(6), 1604-1610.

[7] Topal, A. E., Eren, M. N. & Celik, Y. (2010). Lower extremity arterial injuries over a six-year period: outcomes, risk factors& management. *Vasc. Health Risk Manag.*, *6,*1103-1110.

[8] Olson, S. A. & Glasgow, R. R. (2005). Acute compartment syndrome in lower extremity musculoskeletal trauma. *J. Am. Acad. Orthop. Surg.*, *13*(7), 436-444.

[9] Viegas, S. F., Rimoldi, R., Scarborough, M. & Ballantyne, G. M. (1988). Acute compartment syndrome in the thigh. A case report and a review of the literature. *Clin. Orthop. Relat. Res.* (234), 232-234.

[10] Suzuki, T., Moirmura, N., Kawai, K. & Sugiyama, M. (2005). Arterial injury associated with acute compartment syndrome of the thigh following blunt trauma. *Injury.*, *36*(1), 151-159

[11] Ojike, N. I., Roberts, C. S. & Giannoudis. P. V. (2010). Compartment syndrome of the thigh: a systematic review. *Injury.*, *41*(2), 133-136

[12] McQueen, M. M., Gaston, P. & Court-Brown, C. M. (2000). Acute compartment syndrome. Who is at risk? *J. Bone Joint Surg. Br.*, *82*(2), 200-203

[13] McQueen, M. (1998). Acute compartment syndrome. *Acta Chir. Belg.*, *98*(4), 166-170

[14] Recek, C. (2006). Conception of the venous hemodynamics in the lower extremity. *Angiology.*, *57*(5), 556-563

[15] Wall, C. J., Lynch, J., Harris, I. A., Richardson, M. D., Brand, C., Lowe, A. J. & Sugrue, M. (2010). Liverpool (Sydney) and Royal Melbourne Hospitals. Clinical practice guidelines for the management of acute limb compartment syndrome following trauma. *ANZ J. Surg.*, *80*(3), 151-156

[16] Blasier, R. B. & Pape, J. M. (1991). Simulation of compartment syndrome by rupture of the deep femoral artery from blunt trauma. *Clin. Orthop. Relat. Res.*, (266), 214-217

[17] Mubarak, S. J. & Hargens, A. R. (1983). Acute compartment syndromes. *Surg. Clin. North Am.*, *63*(3), 539-565.

[18] Cohen, M. S., Garfin, S. R., Hargens, A. R. & Mubarak, S. J. (1991). Acute compartment syndrome. Effect of dermotomy on fascial decompression in the leg. *J. Bone Joint Surg. Br.*, *73*(2), 287-290

[19] Maheshwari, R., Taitsman, L. A. & Barei, D. P. (2008). Single-incision fasciotomy for compartmental syndrome of the leg in patients with diaphyseal tibial fractures. *J. Orthop. Trauma.*, *22*(10), 723-730.

[20] Hori, D., Noguchi, K., Nomura, Y., Lefor, A. & Tanaka, H. (2013). Small incision fasciotomy in a patient with compartment syndrome and peripheral arterial occlusive disease. *Ann. Thorac. Cardiovasc. Surg.*, *19*(3), 234-238.

[21] Güler, A., Sahin, M. A., Karabacak, K., Küçükaslan, N., Yokuşoğlu, M. & Tatar, H. (2009). Accompanying embolectomy and closed fasciotomy in the same session for the delayed arterial thromboembolic occlusions in lower extremity. *Anadolu. Kardiyol. Derg.*, *9*(5), 407-410.

[22] Janzing, H. M. & Broos, P. L. (2001). Dermatotraction: an effective technique for the closure of fasciotomy wounds: a preliminary report of fifteen patients. J. *Orthop. Trauma.*, *15*(6), 438-441.

[23] Zannis, J., Angobaldo, J., Marks, M., DeFranzo, A., David, L., Molnar, J. & Argenta, L. (2009). Comparison of fasciotomy wound closures using traditional dressing changes and the vacuum-assisted closure device. *Ann. Plast. Surg.*, *62*(4), 407-409.

[24] Frink, M., Klaus, A. K., Kuther, G., Probst, C., Gosling, T., Kobbe, P., Hildebrand, F., Richter, M., Giannoudis, P. V., Krettek, C. & Pape, H. C. (2007). Long term results of compartment syndrome of the lower limb in polytraumatised patients. *Injury.*, *38*(5), 607-613.

[25] Giannoudis, P. V., Nicolopoulos, C., Dinopoulos, H., Ng, A., Adedapo, S. & Kind, P. (2002). The impact of lower leg compartment syndrome on health related quality of life. *Injury.*, *33*(2), 117-121.

[26] Fitzgerald, A. M., Gaston, P., Wilson, Y., Quaba, A. & McQueen, M. M. (2000).Long-term sequelae of fasciotomy wounds. *Br. J. Plast. Surg.*, *53*(8), 690-693.

[27] Johnson, S. B., Weaver, F. A., Yellin, A. E., Kelly, R. & Bauer, M. (1992). Clinical results of decompressive dermotomy-fasciotomy. *Am. J. Surg.*, *164*(3), 286-290.

[28] Schepsis, A. A., Martini, D. & Corbett, M. (1993). Surgical management of exertional compartment syndrome of the lower leg. Long-term followup. *Am. J. Sports Med.*, *21*(6), 811-817.

[29] Myerson, M. S. (1991). Management of compartment syndromes of the foot. *Clin. Orthop. Relat. Res.*, (*271*), 239-248

In: Compartment Syndrome
Editor: Anna P. Henderson

ISBN: 978-1-63482-831-4

Chapter 6

Paraspinal Compartment Syndrome – An Overview

Ioan Ştefan Florian MD, PhD[*1,3], Magdalena Balaci MD[1] and Lucian Fodor, MD, PhD[2]

[1]Department of Neurosurgery, Emergency County Hospital, Cluj-Napoca, Romania

[2]Department of Plastic Surgery, Emergency County Hospital, Cluj-Napoca, Romania

[3]University of Medicine and Pharmacy 'Iuliu Hatieganu' Cluj-Napoca, Department of Neuroscience

Abstract

Compartment Syndrome is a condition which signifies increased pressure in a confined anatomical space, resulting in compromised circulation and threatening the viability and function of the muscles. The paraspinal region is a potential area for developing compartment syndrome. The erector spinae muscles lay parallel to the dorsolumbar spine and have a curved tube shape, enclosed within a thin fascial layer. The increased intracompartmental pressures produce Paraspinal Compartment Syndrome (PSCS), resulting in the "Bourdon tube effect": the increased intratubal pressure straightens the curved tubes, producing

* Emails Ioan Ştefan Florian – stefanfloriannch@gmail.com

rigidity of the paravertebral muscles and lordosis. Clinical signs include tenderness of the muscles and tenseness; severe pain during the muscle's contractions; and the appearance of pain during passive muscle stretch. Although usually this type of spinal compartment is acute and presents after surgery in this area, it can also become chronic. In chronic conditions, patients might present without any symptoms at rest, exercise-related back pain, a normal range of motion and no neurologic deficit in the lower limbs. This condition is less recognized in clinical practice.

Introduction

Compartment syndrome is "a condition in which increased pressure in a confined anatomical space adversely affects the circulation and threatens the function and viability of tissues therein" [1]. The paraspinal region presents all the anatomical functions and aspects to develop a compartment syndrome in certain instances. The erector spinae muscles can be likened to two curved cylinders enclosed in a fascial system that begins at the nuchal region and ends at the sacrum. Although the compartment syndrome related to the paraspinal muscles is less discussed, its existence has been demonstrated by experimental work and in clinical studies.

Certain instances (trauma, surgery, excessive physical exercise, etc.) can produce a regional increase of pressure, leading to an acute syndrome or the chronic manifestations underlined by Konno et al., [2]. Less discussed is the possibility of triggering paraspinal compartment syndrome (PSCS) after surgery, especially after a posterior approach.

Anatomy of the Paraspinal Region

To better understand the local conditions that can contribute to the development of PSCS, important anatomical elements are described below.

The muscles of the posterior spinal column are divided into three different layers, and have different anatomical aspects according to their region.

Cervical Spine

The superficial muscle layer in the cervical region is the trapezius, which originates in the spinous processes in this region. The middle layer is formed by the splenius capitis. On the lateral part of the splenius capitis are the levator scapulae. The deep layer from the cervical spine is formed by the superficial layer (semispinalis capitis), the middle layer (semispinalis cervicis), and deepest layer (multifidus). On the lateral part of the deep paraspinal muscles lie the longissimus capitis and the longissimus cervicus. The scalene muscles (anterior, middle and posterior) lie anterior to these muscles [3].

The suboccipital triangle of the neck lies between the superior nuchal line from the occiput and the axis (C2), and it is responsible for fine rotation of the head through movements of the atlas and axis.

It is localized deep in the superficial and middle muscle layers from the inferior cervical spine, innervated by the greater occipital and suboccipital nerves.

Both rectus capitis posterior, major and minor, take part of the posterior arch of the atlas and from the spinous process of the axis, and insert into the superior nuchal line.

The obliqus capitis inferior lies between the transverse processes of the atlas and the axis. The obliqus capitis superior originates in the transverse process of the atlas, taking part of of the head rotation and inserts into the superior nuchal line [4].

The platysma, the sternocleidomastoid, the longus coli and the longus capitis muscles are important anatomical landmarks for anterior surgical approaches to the cervical spine.

The blood supply of the cervical spine is provided by the vertebral arteries, branches of the subclavian artery. The costocervical trunk supplies the lower cervical spine [5].

Thoracic and Lumbar Spine

The trapezius represents the superficial layer from the thoracic spine, originating from the cervical spine (ligamentum nuchae) and from the thoracic spine (supraspinous ligament), and is innervated by the spinal accessory nerve. The intermediate layer in the thoracic spine is formed by the rhomboids (the dorsal scapular nerve innervates it) and by the serratus posterior superior muscle.

The latissimus dorsi represents the superficial layer of lumbar spine. Its origins are on the posterior iliac crest, the lower ribs and the lumbodorsal fascia, and it is the thoracodorsal nerve which innervates it.

The intermediate layer of the lumbar spine is represented by the serratus posterior inferior muscle. Its origins are on the lumbar spinous processes for inserting in the ribs [6].

The paraspinal muscles group forms the deep muscle compartment from the thoracic and lumbar spine. This group of muscles runs longitudinally along both sides.

Iliocostalis, longissimus, and spinalis are the paraspinal muscles from the lumbar spine, also called the sacrospinalis or erector spinae muscles. The layer of lumbodorsal fascia has its origins in the supraspinous ligament and iliac spines for travelling laterally in transition to the transversus abdominis fascia (Figure 1).

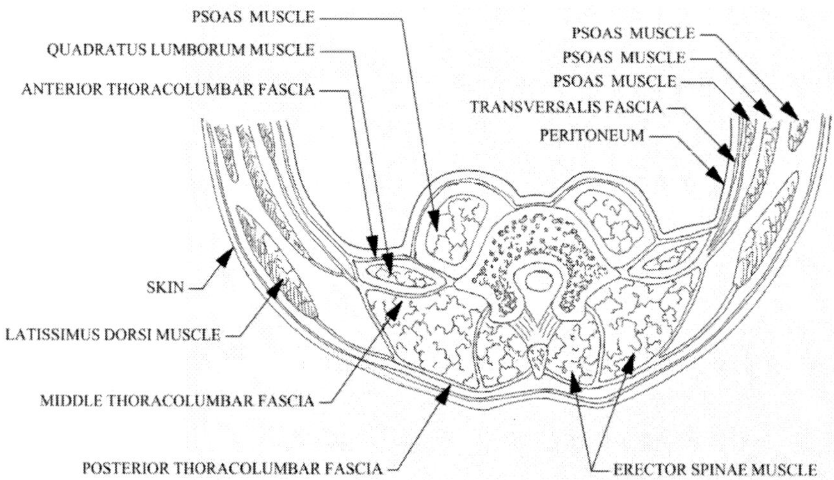

Figure 1. Lumbar compartment.

These muscles travel the thoracic region, and the most median part of the thoracic paraspinal muscles is formed by the: semispinalis (most superficial), multifidus (intermediate layer), and rotators (closest to the skeleton). The paraspinal muscles are supplied by segmental vascular branches from the thoracic and lumbar aorta [7].

The thoracolumbar fascia is a structure that contains several fascia and aponeurotic layers, which separates the paraspinal muscles from the abdominal wall.

The superficial lamina of the posterior thoracolumbar fascia is formed by the serratus posterior inferior and by the aponeurosis of the latissimus dorsi. The paraspinal muscles are surrounded by the deep lamina of the posterior layer of the thoracolumbar fascia (retinacular sheath), which actually acts as a ''hydraulic amplifier'' supporting the lumbosacral spine, and also forms a lumbar interfascial triangle with the posterior and middle layers of the thoracolumbar fascia.

The middle layer of the thoracolumbar fascia (Figure 2) is formed during gestation, between fifth and sixth weeks and is derived from intermuscular septum, separating the epaxial component from the hypaxial musculature.

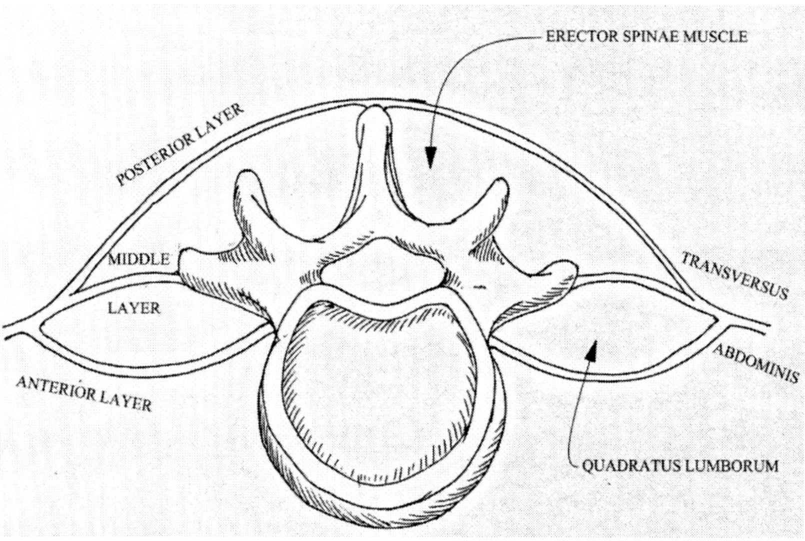

Figure 2. Thoracolumbar fascia - made up of three layers. The anterior layer is the thinnest and the posterior layer is the thickest.

The lateral raphe formed where the sheath crosses the aponeurosis of the transversus abdominis has the role of releasing pressure into the layers of the thoracolumbar fascia from the surrounding muscles. There are two theories about the thoracolumbar fascia [8]:

1) Some authors consider that the paraspinal muscles are surrounded by a continuous fascia attached posteromedially to the spinous processes and anterolaterally to the transverse processes.

2) Others authors consider that the split of the aponeurosis of the transversus abdominis forms the anterior and the posterior walls of the compartment.

Some new studies demonstrate that the continuous sheath that covers the paraspinal muscles has a direct connection with the aponeurosis of the transversus abdominis, which comes from laterally. Even if this aponeurosis seems to take part at the same time to both walls of the paraspinal compartment, some studies showed that most of it forms the anterior wall. It seems that the middle part of the thoracolumbar fascia has two layers, and the compartment is formed by the deep lamina of the posterior layer of the thoracolumbar fascia. During surgical exposure, when it is opened, it presents a lateral boundary which has no indication of splitting [8].

Pathophysiology

For understanding low back pain, it is important to know how these muscles work to influence the stability of the spine and pelvis. Two hypotheses have been described:

1) transfer of the pressure from the thoracolumbar fascia's paraspinal compartment between the posterior and the middle layers of the thoracolumbar fascia (Figure 3);
2) in case of increased tension of the transversus abdominis and internal oblique muscles on the one hand, and incremental pressure from the paraspinal muscle compartment on the other hand, the tension is transmitted to the thoracolumbar fascia.

There is a co-dependent relationship in balancing the tension between the deep abdominal muscles and the lumbar spinal muscles, connected through the aponeurotic components of the thoracolumbar fascia. There is a point (common tendon of the transversus abdominis) where the tension is transmitted between the transversus abdominis muscle, internal oblique muscle and paraspinal muscles [9].

Studies indicate that the thoracolumbar fascia contains nociceptive nerves endings and some injuries of these nerves might produce low back pain. Low back pain can appear also by damaging the muscle's tissues. Immobilization can impair proprioceptive signaling. In producing low back pain injuries of the tissues which are innervated by the same spinal nerves are also incriminated [8].

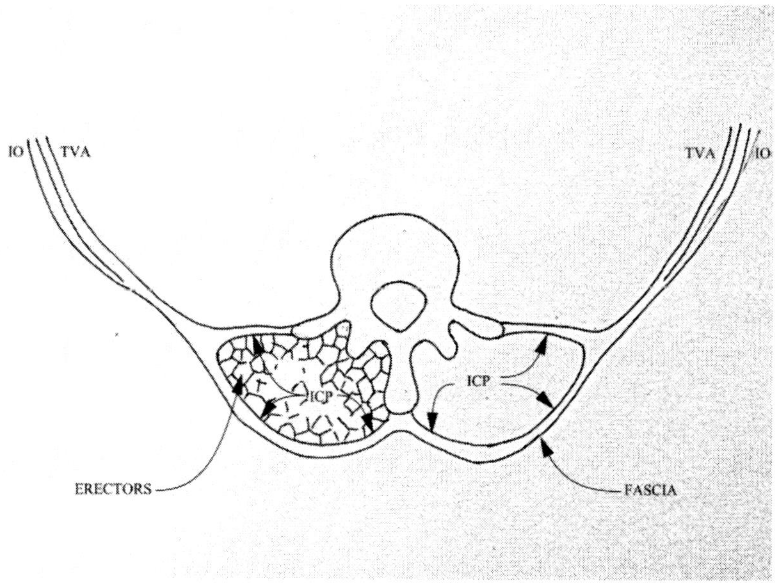

Figure 3. Distribution of increased compartment pressure (ICP=increased compartment pressure, TVA=transversus abdominis, IO=obliqus internus; *drawing by Magdalena Balaci).*

Etiology of PSCS

A compartment syndrome is present when increased pressure causes damage to the muscle, disturbing the neuromuscular functions and local circulation. Some factors described as taking part in developing compartment syndrome are:

- direct trauma to the paraspinal muscle [11]
- a decrease of the vascularization to the paraspinal muscles during aortic surgery, followed by a reperfusion injury [12,13]
- atraumatic acute compartment syndrome [14-16]
- strenuous exercise
- diverse drugs and tonics. The use of isoretinoin [17], steroids [18] and cocaine [19] has been reported to produce muscle damage and

rhabdomyolysis, but there is no evidence to connect substance abuse to developing lumbar PSCS [20].
- several infections, especially postoperative infections (spondylodiscitis)
- endocrine disorders
- electric injuries
- thrombosis of muscular vessels
- peripheral revascularization in case of ischemia [21,22]

The trigger points of low back pain are areas of muscle fascicles which are hyper-contracted and lack energy through impaired function of calcium pumps. This is the mechanism by which back pain occurs: the accumulation of bradykinin and the obstruction of local blood flow [10].

There is a lack of data regarding the appearance of PSCS after trauma. After complex spinal procedures, especially those with large skeletization of the paraspinal muscles, some patients present with low back pain. Styf et al., [23] performed an experimental study to investigate if there is a relation between the external compression and the pressure from the paraspinal compartment during and after lumbar spine surgery. The study included 12 patients who underwent lumbar spine surgery for an average of 271 minutes (range, 90-420 minutes). The pressure was studied as a function of the distance between the retractor blades during surgery [23]. The intramuscular pressure of the bilateral erector spine muscles was measured with the microcapillary infusion technique and three self-retaining retractors were studied – the McCulloch, the Viking and the Richard retractors. The study revealed that the pressure from the paraspinal compartment before surgery was 7.7mm Hg, and varied on the laminas and facet joint levels between 35-69mm Hg. The pressure from the paraspinal compartment varied during surgery between 61-158mm Hg, depending on the distance of the retractor's blades and on which retractor was studied. After surgery, the pressure from the paraspinal compartment never exceeded 30mm Hg at rest. There is a relationship between the intramuscular pressure from the paraspinal compartment and the muscle strain that the blades of the retractors produced during surgery, causing increased intramuscular pressure that might produce muscle ischemia, as reported by Styf et al., [23].

Datta et al., [24] studied 20 patients who underwent decompressive lumbar laminectomy on two levels for lumbar canal stenosis and investigated if there is a relation between the muscle retractors, intramuscular pressure during surgery and back pain and disability after surgery. Two kinds of muscle retractors were studied – the Norfolk-Norwich, and the McCulloch. The intramuscular pressure was measured using a pressure transducer placed in the multifidus muscle and was calculated as a difference between the patient's mean arterial pressure and the intramuscular pressure. The average deep muscle retraction was about 62.7 minutes. Datta et al., [24] made a comparison between the intramuscular pressure during application and after releasing the retractors from the deep muscle during surgery. There was no significant difference concerning intramuscular perfusion pressure between the retractors, but a retraction of more than 60 minutes was associated with back pain and disability. According to the same authors, periodic relaxation of the muscle retractors will contribute to muscle perfusion, thereby reducing postoperative back pain.

Unrecognized as PSCS, most of these patients are subject to various unreliable treatments that may lead to a chronic compartment syndrome [2].

Clinical Signs

The symptoms attributed to PSCS are mainly dominated by pain that is more often described as "an excruciating pain" localized to the paravertebral region. Along with pain, there is a local rigidity of the involved segment with dramatic limitation of movements. Diffuse abdominal tenderness with hypoactive bowel sounds and sensory loss localized in the paraspinal region are considered very important findings in establishing the diagnosis of PSCS [25].

Patients also present localized tenderness and rigidity on the paraspinal region. A pathognomonic sign of acute paraspinal compartment syndrome was considered the localized loss of sensation in the lumbar region. Depending on the involved segment, the patient may also present dyspnea or dysphagia in the cervical region, with the pain radiating from the level of the abdominal wall to the groin, sometimes with paralytic ileus [25].

According to Nathan [20], patients with acute PSCS present with excruciating low back pain, without any history of this type of pain, radiating or not, within 12 hours from the incident.

According to Konno [2], important signs for chronic compartment syndrome are:

- no symptoms at rest
- normal range of motion
- low back pain during exercise
- improvement on extension
- no neurological deficit in the lower extremities

Diagnostic Work-Up

A history of trauma, surgical intervention on the spine or on the major thoracic or abdominal vessels, endovascular treatment, heavy physical exercise, in a context of symptoms presented before, must raise the possibility of developing PSCS [23, 24]. In order to obtain optimal treatment, diagnosis is the key, whether acute or chronic PSCS.

The laboratory tests of the patients who presented with acute paraspinal compartment syndrome revealed:

- rhabdomyolysis due to muscle damage
- increased level of creatinine phosphokinase (CPK) (more than 2000-40000UI/L) and serum glutamic-oxaloacetic transaminase (SGOT)
- increased serum myoglobin
- increased urine myoglobin

Intramuscular pressure is increased (70-80mmHg). Intramuscular pressure measurements are useful in diagnosing paraspinal compartment syndrome. Although there are some differences among the models used for measuring intramuscular pressure, the main tool is represented by a beveled 18-gauge needle connected to a pressure transducer. The needle is inserted into the muscular compartment. Then, less than 3/10cc of saline is injected into the muscle. After a few seconds, equilibrium will be reached and the pressure can be recorded. There is some controversy regarding the time until irreversible ischemic changes appear and at what pressure the infraction is present. Sheridan et al., [26] studied 22 patients who were treated within 12 hours from the incident and reported a 68% rate of recovery to normal function. Only 8% of the patients treated after 12 hours from the incident were able to return to normal function [27].

An intramuscular pressure of 30-50mm Hg is necessary to produce ischemia, while normal pressure is between 3-8mmHg [19, 20]. The intramuscular compartment measurements should be used only to confirm the clinical diagnosis and should not be used as a screening procedure for those who are at risk for developing compartment syndrome [27]. Technetium Tc 99 m bone scan is very helpful in assessing the extent of muscle damage [12, 28, 29].

Imaging diagnosis is mainly based on MRI examination. The most frequent finding is edema noted as a homogenous signal in T2-weighted images. On the follow-up program, muscle atrophy could be also seen [17].

Treatment

Identifying this syndrome in the acute phase (immediately after trauma or surgical intervention) or in the chronic stages would permit the establishment of an adequate attitude to decrease the pressure in the involved paraspinal region. At the same time, it would allow for the avoidance of multiple and improper treatment methods that might not just impede the patient's recovery, but also aggravate the condition.

A debate regarding the most effective treatment, conservative or surgical, is ongoing in the literature. Regarding conservative treatment, administration of crystalloid fluid infusions, urine alkalization, bed rest, analgesics, opioids, and sedatives are the usual therapeutic measures recommended for the condition. Usually, patients returned to baseline function with conservative treatment in four to six month; however, they tended to have chronic back pain on physical activities [25].

Karram et al., [30] reported a case of hyperbaric oxygen therapy's efficiency for the treatment of an acute exertional PSCS. The use of hyperbaric oxygen therapy improved tissue viability by oxygen delivery to ischemic areas [31]. The levels of creatine kinase started to decrease coincident with the initiation of hyperbaric oxygen therapy, and the pain improved after up to 36 hours of hyperbaric oxygen therapy [31]. The hyperbaric oxygen therapy is a useful tool in the treatment of acute exertional PSCS, in case of a clear diagnosis. It improves the pain and reduces the creatine kinase values, without disturbing renal function [23].

Special attention must to be paid to prevent development of PSCS after spinal surgery. Gentle skeletization with isolation and dissection of muscle insertion on the bones, avoiding excessive use of cautery with high power, meticulous hemostasis of the paravertebral muscles, and avoidance of a too tight closure of the fascial layer at the end of the procedure are some important steps to prevent PSCS. Severe local pain in the immediate postoperative period is a sign of the possible development of PSCS. Immediate MRI examination is mandatory to rule out local complications. In the presence of a large hematoma and diffuse edema in the muscles, immediate surgical exploration is the best solution, with evacuation of the hematoma and/or fasciotomy. Severe back pain in 3-4 weeks after a spinal procedure can be a sign of local infection. MRI examination is the most reliable diagnostic tool. The presence of local edema in the adjacent vertebrae with unhomogeneous enhancement in the muscles and region is a direct sign of spondylodiscitis. Usually, intravenous administration of antibiotics is not enough; reopening with clearance of the surgical field followed by local washing with antibiotic and antiseptic solution for 3 to 5 days will solve the complication. Bed rest up to the disappearance of pain generated by movement, opioids, and maintenance of antibiotic therapy up to six weeks are supplementary methods based on our experience.

According to experience with surgical treatment of compartment syndrome in other locations, it seems that fasciotomy (unilateral or bilateral) is the treatment of choice for PSCS. Khan et al., [25] performed a bilateral fasciotomy in the case they published. After surgery, the pressure returned to normal (<10mmHg) and the level of creatine kinase decreased significantly; no complications appeared after surgery, except a wound seroma that resolved after six aspirations. Within a month, the patient did not complain of any back pain and he returned to sporting activities [25]. Similar procedures were performed by other authors [14-16] to treat PSCS.

Related to surgery of the spine, it is crucial to avoid both extensive dissection and damage of the paraspinal muscles and very tight sutures in this region. These elements represent probable causes for persistent low back pain as a result of PSCS. Minimally invasive surgery may prove to be the key in avoiding the development of paraspinal compartment syndrome.

Conclusion

From the data in the literature, we can conclude that PSCS is a present but under-diagnosed entity. This diagnosis should be considered when a patient presents with excruciating localized back pain following exertion, downhill skiing or surfing, direct trauma or post-surgery. Increased pain on flexion that is relieved on extension with no prior history of back pain indicates a possible PSCS. On local examination, usually there is bilateral or unilateral paraspinal muscle rigidity, with diffuse abdominal tenderness, along with localized sensory alteration in the paraspinal region.

Most relevant investigation is elevated CPK, elevated SGOT, and myoglobinuria. On MRI there is an increase in signal intensity inside the compartment. In cases of doubt, measured intramuscular pressure (70–80mm Hg) is the method to confirm the diagnosis [20]. Surgical fasciotomy is the recommended treatment in emergency, once the diagnosis is firmly established. Otherwise, bad rest, crystalloid infusion, opioids and urine alkalinisation to prevent renal failure are conservative measures with variable results. Prevention is important in spine surgery, minimal invasiveness and gentle maneuvers on the paraspinal muscles being the key elements.

References

[1] *Stedman's Medical Dictionary*, 27th edition, Philadelphia, Lippincot Williams & Wilkins, pp175 (2000).

[2] S. Konno, S. Kikuchi, and N. Yoshihiro. The relationship between intramuscular pressure of the paraspinal muscles and low back pain. *Spine*. 19(19), 2186-2189 (1994).

[3] J. German, et al. Spine Surgery: The cervical spine and cervicothoracic junction, in: *Spine Surgery: Techniques, Complication Avoidance, and Management*, 2nd edition. E. C. Benzel, editor, Philadelphia: Elsevier Inc (2005).

[4] R. McGuire and A. Ragab. Spine Surgery: occipital cervical region, in: *Spine Surgery: Techniques, Complication Avoidance, and Management*, 2nd edition. E. C. Benzel, editor, Philadelphia: Elsevier Inc (2005).

[5] H. Crock and H. Yoshizawa. *The Blood Supply of the Vertebral Column and Spinal Cord in Man*. New York: Springer-Verlag (1977).

[6] W. Parke, C. Bono and S. Garfin. The Spine: Applied anatomy of the spine, in: *The Spine*, 5th edition, Volume 1. H. N. Herkowitz, R. H. Rothman and F. A. Simeone, editors. Philadelphia: Saunders Elsevier (2006).

[7] S. Hoppenfeld, P. DeBoer and R. Hutton. Surgical exposures in orthopaedics: the anatomic approach, in: *The Spine*, 4th edition. Philadelphia: Lippincott Williams &Wilkins (2009).

[8] F. H. Willard, A. Vleeming, M. D. Schuenke, L. Danneels and R. Schleip. The thoracolumbar fascia: anatomy, function and clinical considerations. *J. Anat.* 221(6), 507-536 (2012).

[9] Vleeming, M. D. Schuenke, L. Danneels and F. H. Willard. The functional coupling of the deep abdominal and paraspinal muscles: the effects of simulated paraspinal muscle contraction on force transfer to the middle and posterior layer of the thoracolumbar fascia. *J. Anat* 225, 447-462 (2014).

[10] D. G. Simons. Myofascial pain syndromes. where we are? Where are we going? *Arch. Phys. Med. Rehabil.* 69(3 Pt 1), 207-212 (1988).

[11] J. Sava, A. Moelleken and K. Waxman. Cardiac arrest caused by reperfusion injury after lumbar paraspinal compartment syndrome. *J. Trauma*. 46, 196-197 (1999).

[12] J. Ferreira, C. Galle, A. Aminian, P. Michael, S. Guyot, J. P. De Wilde, S. Motte, J. C. Wautrecht and J. P. Dereume. Lumbar paraspinal rabdomyolisis and compartment syndrome after abdominal aortic aneurysm repair. *J. Vasc. Surg*. 37, 198-201 (2003).

[13] N. Osamura, K. Takahashi, M. Endo, H. Kurumaya and I. Shima. Lumbar paraspinal myonecrosis after abdominal vascular surgery: a case report. *Spine*. 25, 1852-1854 (2000).

[14] D. Carr, L. Gilbertson, J. Frymoyer, M. Krag and M. Pope. Lumbar paraspinal compartments syndrome. A case report with physiologic and anatomic studies. *Spine*. 10, 816-820 (1985).

[15] F. A. DiFazio, R. A. Barth and J. W. Frymoyer. Acute lumbar paraspinal compartment syndrome. A case report. *J. Bone Joint Surg. Am*. 73, 1101-1103 (1991).

[16] Kitajima, S. Tachibana, Y. Hirota and K. Nakamichi. Acute paraspinal compartment syndrome treated with surgical decompression: a case report. *Am. J. Sports Med*. 30, 283-285 (2002).

[17] L. Wik, J. M. Patterson and A. E. Oswald. Exertional paraspinal muscle rhabdomyolysis and compartment syndrome: a cause of back pain not to be missed. *Clin. Rheumatol*. 29, 803–805 (2010).

[18] U. Farkash, N. Shabshin and M. Pritsch Perry. Rhabdomyolysis of the deltoid muscle in a bodybuilder using anabolic-androgenic steroids: a case report. J. *Athl. Train*. 44, 98–100 (2009).

[19] P. Singhal, B. Horowitz, M. C. Quinones, M. Sommer, M. Faulkner and M. Grosser. Acute renal failure following cocaine abuse. *Nephron*. 52, 76–78 (1989).

[20] S. Nathan, C. S. Roberts and D. Deliberato. Lumbar paraspinal compartment syndrome. *Int. Orthop*. 36, 1221–1227 (2012).

[21] R. Vanholder, M. S. Sever, E. Erek and N. Lameire. Rhabdomyolysis. *J. Am. Soc. Nephrol*. 11, 1553-1561 (2000).

[22] M. S. Slater and R. J. Mullins. Rhabdomyolysis and myoglobinuric renal failure in trauma and surgical patients: a review. *J. Am. Coll. Surg*. 186, 693-716 (1998).

[23] R. Styf and J. Willién. The effects of external compression by three different retractors on pressure in the erector spine muscles during and after posterior lumbar spine surgery in humans. *Spine*. (Phila Pa 1976) 23(3), 354-358 (1998).

[24] G. Datta, K. K. Gnanalingham, D. Peterson, N. Mendoza, K. O'Neill, J. Van Dellen, A. McGregor and S. P. Hughes SP. Back pain and disability after lumbar laminectomy: is there a relationship to muscle retraction? *Neurosurgery*. 54(6), 1413-1420 (2004).

[25] R. J. Khan, D. P. Fick, C. A. Guier, M. J. Menolascino and M. C. Neal. Acute paraspinal compartment syndrome. A case report. *J. Bone Joint Surg. Am*. 87(5), 1126-1128 (2005).

[26] G. W. Sheridan and F. A. Matsen 3rd. Fasciotomy in the treatment of the acute compartment syndrome. *J. Bone Joint Surg. Am.* 58(1), 112-115 (1976).

[27] M. R. Garner, S. A. Taylor, E. Gausden and J. P. Lyden. Compartment syndrome: diagnosis, management, and unique concerns in the twenty-first century. *HSS. J.* 10(2), 143-152 (2014).

[28] P. A. Frymoyer, R. Giammarco, F. M. Farrar and E. T. Schroeder. Technetium Tc 99m medronate bone scanning in rhabdomyolysis. *Arch. Intern. Med*. 145, 1991-1995 (1985).

[29] T. Mochizuki, W. N. Tauxe and J. A. Perper. Technetium-99m MDP scintigraphy of rhabdomyolysis induced exertional heat stroke: a case report. *Ann. Nucl. Med.* 4, 111-113 (1990).

[30] M. D. Karam, A. Amendola and S. Mendoza-Lattes. Case report: successful treatment of acute exertional paraspinal compartment syndrome with hyperbaric oxygen therapy. *Iowa Orthop. J.* 30, 188-190 (2010).

[31] E. Greensmith. Hyperbaric oxygen therapy in extremity trauma. *J. Am. Acad. Orthop. Surg*. 12, 376-384 (2004).

In: Compartment Syndrome
Editor: Anna P. Henderson

ISBN: 978-1-63482-831-4

Chapter 7

Orbital Compartment Syndrome in Sphenoidal Wing Neurosurgical Procedures. Literature Review

Ioan Ştefan Florian MD, PhD*[*1,3], Cristian Kakucs MD[1] and Lucian Fodor, MD, PhD[2]

[1]Department of Neurosurgery, Emergency County Hospital, Cluj-Napoca, Romania

[2]Department of Plastic Surgery, Emergency County Hospital, Cluj-Napoca, Romania

[3]University of Medicine and Pharmacy 'Iuliu Hatieganu' Cluj-Napoca, Department of Neuroscience

Abstract

Orbital compartment syndrome (OCS) is a rare but treatable ophthalmic surgical emergency, caused most often by a retrobulbar hematoma, facial trauma being the most frequent etiological factor. Iatrogenic causes are rarely discussed, and are most often overlooked.

[*] Emails: Ioan Ştefan Florian – stefanfloriannch@gmail.com

The prone position in long surgical procedures, such as posterior fossa or spinal surgery, has been recognized in the literature, but intracranial surgery for vascular or tumoral lesions along the sphenoid wing is rarely presented as an etiological factor for this frightening complication. Irreversible blindness can occur if the lateral canthotomy is not performed urgently. Multiple surgical procedures that can produce OCS are described in the literature. OCS can occur after endoscopic sinus surgery, transorbital neuroendoscopic surgery, cerebral aneurysm surgery, embolization of arterio-venous malformation or carotid-cavernous fistula, or any procedure performed in anterior skull base surgery.

It is for these reasons that we offer a comprehensive review of the orbital compartment syndrome from a neurosurgical point of view, focusing especially on neurosurgical procedures around the sphenoidal wing. We will not refer to lesions that secondarily involve the orbit, but will focus on those surgeries that address intracranial pathologies (vascular, tumoral or malformative), having OCS as a potential complication. Anatomical relationships, surgical procedures, possible pathophysiological mechanisms, clinical presentation and management of OCS are presented, based on actual literature and personal experience.

Recognition of OCS in the immediate postoperative period is of the outmost importance considering that, untreated, this complication may lead to visual loss. By being aware of the possible occurrence of OCS and by performing a relatively simple surgical procedure (canthotomy), blindness can be avoided.

1. Introduction

The Orbital Compartment Syndrome (OCS) is an ophthalmological emergency produced by an acute increase of orbital pressure that subsequently leads to hypoperfusion of critical neural structures confined in the limited space of the orbit. This condition may lead to visual loss and ophtahlmoplegia that are irreversible if not recognized and treated in an emergency situation [1, 2]. The most frequent cause of OCS is retrobulbar hematoma, facial trauma usually being involved as an etiological factor, with iatrogenic factors less discussed in the literature. In this chapter we will underline the relevant anatomy, pathophysiology, clinical presentation, and neurosurgical procedures that could lead to OCS in order to recognize and apply the proper treatment to this pathology, frequently neglected by neurosurgeons.

2. Relevant Anatomy of the Orbit

The orbit is divided into two main components: the bony orbit and the elements inside the bony orbit.

The orbit is a conical structure composed of irregular walls surrounding the vision body, and muscles, vessels and nerves that are around the globe. The average volume of an orbit is about $30cm^3$. Orbit height is about 35mm and width around 40mm. The length of the orbit is 45mm if measured from the medial edge of the base levels orbit to the orbital apex, while the length from the edge side to the orbital apex is less than about 10mm [3, 4].

The orbit presents four walls, four edges, an apex and a base. The orbit is made up of seven bones: the orbital process of the frontal bone, the lesser and greater wings of the sphenoid bone, the orbital facet of the maxillary bone, the orbital facet of the zygomatic bone, the orbital part of the palatine bone's orbital process, the lateral surface of the lacrimal bone, and the lateral surface of the ethmoid bone [5-7] (Figure 1).

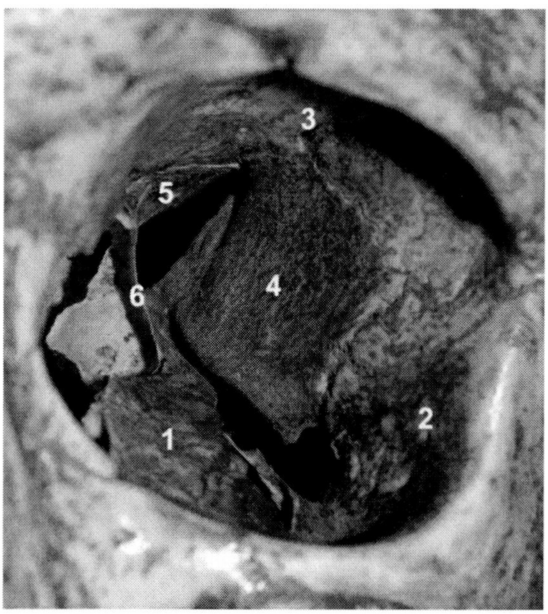

Figure 1. The bony orbit. 1 - Maxillar bone; 2 - Zygomatic bone; 3 - Frontal bone; 4 - Greater wing of the sphenoid bone; 5 - Lesser wing of the sphenoid bone; 6 - Ethmoidal bone (photo by Cristian Kakucs).

Anatomical elements contained in the orbit.

- nervous elements represented by the ciliary ganglion and the nerves: optic, oculomotor, trochlear, frontal, lacrimal, abducens and nasociliar;
- vascular elements represented by the ophthalmic artery and its subdivisions and the superior and inferior ophtalmic veins;
- extrinsic muscles and intrinsic muscles;
- eyeball;
- ligaments: suspensory ligament of the eyeball, Whitnall ligament and the suspensory ligament Lockwood [8];
- intraorbital fat;
- lacrimal gland and naso-lacrimal canal.

The ophthalmic artery arises from the supraclinoidian segment of the internal carotid artery, passes inferior and lateral to the optic nerve, and represents the main vascular axis of the orbit (Figure 2). The ophthalmic artery has the following branches: lacrimal artery, central retinal artery, ciliary arteries, anterior ethmoidal artery, posterior ethmoidal artery, supraorbital artery and suborbital artery [3, 4].

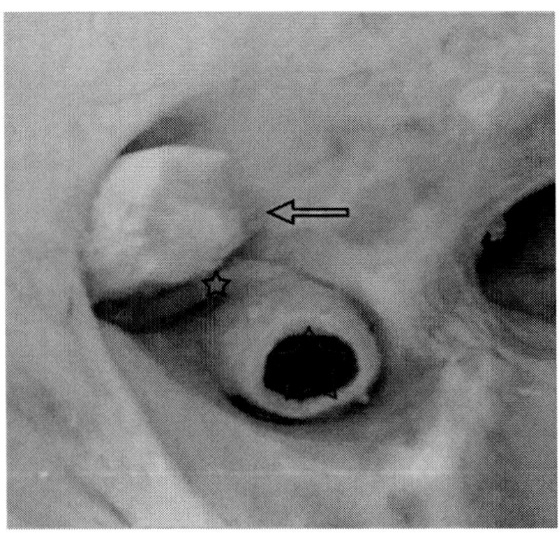

Figure 2. The ophthalmic artery. Red star - internal carotid artery; black star – ophthalmic artery; black arrow – optic nerve (photo by Cristian Kakucs).

The extrinsic muscles of the eyeball mainly originate at the level of the Zinn tendinous ring and form the muscle cone.

Fissures and Orbital Foramens

Superior Orbital Fissure

The superior orbital fissure is located near the orbital apex and is crossed by the oculomotor nerve, trochlear nerve, abducens nerve, the ophthalmic branch of the trigeminal nerve and the superior ophthalmic vein [6].

Inferior Orbital Fissure

The inferior orbital fissure is located about 10mm from the infero-lateral orbital rim and links the pterigo-palatine fossa to the lower portion of the orbit. This fissure is bordered laterally by the zygomatic and sphenoid bones, while the medial border is represented by the maxilla and the zygomatic arch. [6].

Optic Canal

The optic canal is located medial to the superior orbital fissure at the level of the orbital apex. It has a diameter of about 5mm and a length not exceeding 10mm. The edges are completely composed of the sphenoid bone. The optic canal is separated from the superior orbital fissure by the optic strut. This canal is passed by the optic nerve and the ophthalmic artery [3].

The orbit is limited anteriorly by tarsal plates and their medial and lateral insertions, the globe covered by conjunctiva. The canthi are the anatomic junction of the upper and lower lids at the both extremities. The orbit communicates directly with the cranial cavity, frontal sinus, sphenoidal sinus, maxillary sinus, ethmoidal sinus, temporal region, infratemporal region and anterior region of the face through the mentioned fissures and foramens [4, 6].

3. Epidemiology

Orbital compartment syndrome is a rare pathological entity that occurs after a facial trauma or after surgery on the orbit or the adjacent structures. OCS occurs at a rate of about 2-3% in facial trauma patients, according to the literature [9]. The real incidence seems to be higher, but not all cases are properly recognized and reported [1, 10]. There are even poorer data regarding OCS after neurosurgical procedures and only a few cases are reported in the literature [11, 12]. In reality, nobody knows the real incidence of OCS, but it seems to be higher than that reported in the literature. Concerning OCS related to neurosurgical procedures along the sphenoid wing, there are only a few reports in the literature. Some surgeons are less familiar with OCS because it is less recognized and, consequently, less reported.

4. Etiology

OCS can be caused by many intraorbital, intracranial or extracranial pathologies. The most common cause of developing OCS is retrobulbar hematoma, frequently caused by facial injuries. Other causes of occurrence of this pathological entity could include: tumors, blood dyscrasias, intraocular infection, prolonged hypoxemia, inflammation, foreign body, venous thrombosis and emphysema [13, 14].

There are a number of invasive procedures that can produce OCS. Among the most common are: endoscopic sinus surgery, transorbital neuroendoscopic surgery (TONES), cerebral aneurysms surgery, embolization of carotid-cavernous fistula or arteriovenous malformations [11, 12, 15]. In theory, any invasive procedure on the anterior cranial fossa may lead to retrobulbar hematoma or intraorbital edema having, as a consequence, increased intraorbital pressure that may lead to OCS.

Transorbital neuroendoscopy is a relatively new surgical technique that aims to add new surgical corridors for the frontal sinus, orbit and anterior cranial fossa. Using this technique, TONES can treat various pathologies, such as epidural abscesses, orbital abscesses, fronto-orbital mucocele or subperiosteal abscesses [3]. Endoscopic sinus surgery can cause a number of ophthalmic complications, including OCS. Published data suggest the occlusion of the central retinal artery due to fat embolism as the mechanism of developing OCS [16]. Sia et al., [17] described the case of a 69-year old patient who presented with OCS after transvenous embolization of a carotid-cavernous fistula. The mechanism of the OCS was the thrombosis of the superior ophthalmic vein. Even though thrombosis of the superior ophthalmic vein is a rare complication after carotid-cavernous fistula embolization, it may cause a compartment syndrome leading to permanent visual deficits. Canthotomy and cantholisis were performed and the outcome was favorable without any visual sequelae after this event [17].

Very few cases of OCS following brain surgery have been reported in the medical literature. The outcomes were variable and depended on the speed of the diagnosis and that of the surgery [12-18]. Apart from invasive procedures that can produce OCS, another cause might be the head position during surgical intervention. The compartment syndrome may occur in the prone position [19], due to improper positioning with compression of the eyeballs in long-lasting procedures [1].

5. Pathophysiology

The orbital space is a closed space, which is why an acute increase in pressure at this level can cause compartment syndrome. The physiological intraocular pressure is between 10 and 20mmHg [2, 14, 20] and the intraorbital pressure is between 3 and 6mmHg [21]. Usually, the main mechanism leading to the development of OCS is an acute increase of intraorbital pressure causing decreased perfusion which leads to ischemia, as can be seen in other compartment syndromes [20]. An acute increase in intraorbital pressure (above 20mmHg) lasting more than 60-100 minutes causes irreversible visual damage, so this syndrome must be quickly recognized and surgery must be performed as quickly as possible to avoid irreversible visual damage and complete ophthalmoplegia [14, 20, 22]. Intraocular and intraorbital pressure increases immediately after a hemorrhage in the retrobular space because of the lack of distensibility [14].

Ischemia of the optic nerve can occur if the vasa nervosum is affected by the increased intraorbital pressure. Also, increased intraorbital pressure can produce retinal ischemia which occurs when the central retinal artery is affected by increased pressure in the retrobulbar space [14].

There are multiple mechanisms that lead to increased intraocular pressure, which vary depending on the etiology of the compartment syndrome, but these can all lead to irreversible loss of vision [2]. Even though several pathophysiological mechanisms that can produce this syndrome have been taken into consideration, they still are not completely understood. The main mechanisms of occurrence of this syndrome include local hypoperfusion and swelling of intraorbital structures. Some studies also incriminate arterial vasospasm that may arise from injury. All these mechanisms produce an increase in intraorbital pressure and automatically produce an increase in intraocular pressure. Local hypoperfusion appears due to compression of the central retinal artery and other vessels that supply the muscular-nervous elements of the orbit. One study showed that retinal changes can appear after injecting experimentally just 7ml of fluid into the orbit [23]. All these pathophysiological mechanisms lead to the formation of irreversible neurological damage if surgery is not performed immediately [24].

6. Clinical Signs

From a clinical point of view, OCS may present as swelling and congestion of the periorbital region, ecchymosis, proptosis and ophthalmoplegia [11, 12]. In addition to these complaints that may be present in OCS, increased intraocular pressure is also present [2, 17]. Of the many injuries that occur as a result of these mechanisms, blindness is certainly the most feared complication of this syndrome.

7. OCS in Neurosurgery

The occurrence of this syndrome following neurosurgical intervention performed along the sphenoid wing is due to the proximity to the orbit and to the risk of damaging vascular elements entering the orbit. Rarely, OCS may cause blindness after neurosurgical intervention for a vascular disease, such as brain aneurysm or arterio-venous malformations [12]. The first case of compartment syndrome after resection of a frontal cerebral arterio-venous malformation described in literature was in 2014. The second case was secondary to embolization of a dural arterio-venous malformation from the skull base. After surgery, the patients had unilateral blindness, proptosis, complete ophthalmoplegia, chemosis and increased intraocular pressure. Both patients were left with postoperative unilateral blindness [11, 15].

In brain aneurysm surgery, there are a few cases described in the literature for developing OCS secondary to surgery. In one such case [15], postoperative bilateral blindness and complete ophtahlmoplegia occurred immediately. A bifrontal approach to solve the cerebral aneurysm was performed. The risk factors convicted in the mechanisms of developing OCS were direct eye pressure caused by local skin flap and congestion caused by head positioning. Fourteen hours after surgery, the patient developed bilateral chemosis and proptosis and it was decided to perform canthotomy and cantolysis but without satisfactory results, and the patient remained with bilateral blindness [15]. In another reported case of cerebral aneurysm [12], the patient presented after surgery with OCS. Lateral canthotomy and superior cantholysis was performed immediately. After the surgical and medical treatment, the patient's outcome was good with partial resolution of the symptoms [12].

Despite the fact that neurosurgical procedures are scarcely presented in the literature as a cause of OCS, we consider it necessary to underline certain aspects. Some neurosurgical approaches have a high potential to produce a retro-orbital hematoma. One of the most frequently used in aneurismal surgery is the pterional approach, described by Yasargil [25]. A proper placement of the so called "key hole" will open simultaneously the intracranial compartment and the orbit, creating the condition for a retrobulbar hematoma during a surgical procedure. Other surgical procedures, such as the Fronto-Orbito-Zigomatic (FTOZ) approach, extradural drilling of the sphenoid wing, and anterior clinoid, may create conditions for the development of OCS.

Additionally, postoperative local edema, swelling and oozing may increase intraorbital pressure in the immediate postoperative period. We must be aware of all these aspects in order to closely follow a patient's visual impairment and to act accordingly to prevent the development of OCS.

8. Treatment of OCS

OCS is a surgical emergency and should be recognized quickly so as not to reach irreversible visual deficits. The gold standard of OCS treatment is lateral canthotomy and inferior cantholysis. This procedure involves cutting the lateral canthal tendon toward the orbital rim, dissection and catting the inferior limb of the tendon from the bony orbit (Figure 3).

Lateral canthotomy associated with inferior cantholysis represent the most effective decompression methods of the orbit as they lower intraocular pressure [26]. This relief procedure should be performed as quickly as possible. The literature data shows that patients with OCS who undergo orbital decompression within two hours of its occurrence fully recover, while patients who underwent decompression after 4-6 hours presented different degrees of visual impairment [27]. All patients with a history and clinical signs of compartment syndrome should undergo canthotomy and cantholysis as soon as possible, in order to minimize the risk of visual deficits [27].

Several versions of orbital decompression are described in the literature: lower orbital septum release or removal of the orbital bone structures. The latter option is more difficult to perform because it takes time and the patient must be in the operating room. However, the first intervention (inferior orbital septum release) can be achieved even at the bedside, which is a major advantage [24, 26].

Lateral canthotomy is a simple surgical procedure that should be performed by any neurosurgeon if the patient developed OCS after a neurosurgical operation [11]. Lateral canthotomy in the setting of OCS is a emergency maneuver similar to that of external ventricular drainage in acute hydrocephalus [29]. After lateral canthotomy and inferior cantholysis, other more extensive surgical techniques can be performed, if the initial one does not give satisfactory results.

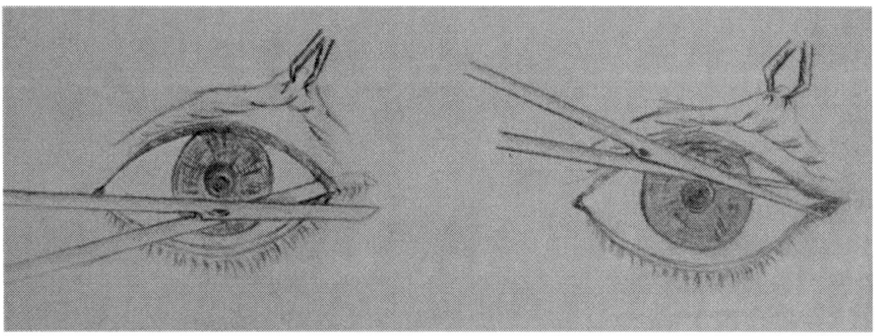

Figure 3. Lateral cantholysis (drawing by Cristian Kakucs)

9. Outcome in OCS

The outcome of orbital compartment syndrome depends on the immediate recognition and treatment of this entity. Lateral canthotomy and inferior cantholysis are mandatory requirements if we have to treat OCS; otherwise, blindness is inevitable.

In addition to lateral canthotomy and inferior cantholysis, other methods are described in the literature, such as osmotic agents and corticosteroids. Regardless of the medication we use or of other adjuvant therapy, the fact remains that only canthotomy and cantolisis decrease intraocular pressure and, thus, allow for the remission of visual symptoms in the orbital compartment syndrome [1, 14].

References

[1] V. Lima, B. Burt, I. Leibovitch, V. Prabhakaran, R. A. Goldberg and D. Selva, Orbital compartment syndrome: the ophthalmic surgical emergency. *Surv. Ophthalmol.* 54(4), 441-449 (2009).

[2] F. Haubner, H. Jägle, D. P. Nunes, S. Schleder, N. Cvetkova, T. Kühnel T and H.G. Gassner, Orbital compartment: effects of emergent canthotomy and cantholysis. *Eur. Arch. Otorhinolaryngol.* 272(2), 479-483 (2015).

[3] H. W. Richard, *Youmans Neurological Surgery*, 6th edition, Elsevier Saunders, 2, pp1655 (2011).

[4] L. Rhoton, *Cranial anatomy and surgical approaches*, Lippincott Williams & Wilkins pp331-349 (2003).

[5] T. A. Turvey and B. A. Golden, Orbital anatomy for the surgeon. *Oral Maxillofac. Surg. Clin. North Am.* 24(4), 525–536 (2012).

[6] S. F. Abed, P. Shams, S. Shen, P. J. Adds, J. M. Uddin and M. Manisali, A cadaveric study of the cranio-orbital foramen and its and its significance in orbital surgery. *Plast. Reconstr. Surg.* 129(2), 307e-311e (2012).

[7] C. Martins, I. E. Costa e Silva, A. Campero, A. Yasuda, L. R. Aguiar, M. Tatagiba and A. Rhoton Jr, *Microsurgical Anatomy of the Orbit: The Rule of Seven*, Anatomy Research International, 2011, Article ID 468727 (2011).

[8] P. N. Manson, C. M. Clifford, C. T. Su, N. T. Iliff and R. Morgan R, Mechanisms of global support and posttraumatic enophthalmos: I. The anatomy of the ligament sling and its relation to intramuscular cone orbital fat. *Plast. Reconstr. Surg.* 77, 193–202 (1986)/

[9] G. R. Holt and J. E. Holt, Incidence of eye injuries in facial fractures: an analysis of 727 cases. *Otolaryngol. Head Neck Surg.* 91(3), 276-279 (1983).

[10] E. Oester Jr, B. T. Fowler and J. C. Fleming, Inferior orbital septum release compared with lateral canthotomy and cantholysis in the management of orbital compartment syndrome. *Ophthal. Plast. Reconstr. Surg.* 28(1), 40-43 (2012).

[11] M. H. Levin, H. E. Moss, S. L. Pineles, L. J. Bagley, G. G. Heuer, E. L. Zager, L. J. Balcer, S. L. Galetta and M. R. Vagefi, Orbital congestion complicating treatment of cerebral vascular anomalies. *World Neurosurg.* 82(1-2), 239.e13-7 (2014).

[12] J. Gauden, T. Hardy, H. G. Mack, H. V. Danesh-Meyer and A. H. Kaye, Orbital compartment syndrome following aneurysm surgery. *J. Clin. Neurosci.* 19(7), 1032–1036 (2012).

[13] E. J. Wladis, T. R. Peebles and D. A. Weinberg, Management of acute orbital hemorrhage with obstruction of the ophthalmic artery during attempted coil embolization of a dural arteriovenous fistula of the cavernous sinus. *Ophthal. Plast. Reconstr. Surg.* 23, 57–59 (2007).

[14] D. Rowh, J. W. Ufberg, T. C. Chan, G. M. Vilke and R. A. Harrigan. Lateral canthotomy and cantholysis: Emergency management of orbital compartment syndrome. *J. Emerg. Med.* 2014 Dec 15. pii: S0736-4679(14)01222-0. doi: 10.1016/j.jemermed.2014.11.002. [Epub ahead of print].

[15] Y. Takahashi, H. Kakizaki, D. Selva and I. Leibovitch. Bilateral orbital compartment syndrome and blindness after cerebral aneurysm repair surgery. *Ophthal. Plast. Reconstr. Surg.* 26, 299–301 (2010).

[16] K. E. Kim, S. J. Ahn, S. J. Woo, N. Kim and J. M. Hwang. Central retinal artery occlusion caused by fat embolism following endoscopic sinus surgery. *J. Neuroophthalmol.* 33(2), 149-150 (2013).

[17] P. I. Sia, D. I. Sia, R. Scroop and D. Selva D. Orbital compartment syndrome following transvenous embolization of carotid-cavernous fistula. *Orbit.* 33(1), 52-54 (2014).

[18] S. R. Ballard, R. W. Enzenauer, T. O'Donnell, J. C. Fleming, G. Risk and A. N. Waite. Emergency lateral canthotomy and cantholysis: a simple procedure to preserve vision from sight threatening orbital hemorrhage. *J. Spec. Oper. Med.* 9(3), 26-32 (2009).

[19] Leibovietch, R. Casson, C. Laforest and D. Selva. Ischemic orbital compartment syndrome as a complication of spinal surgery in the prone position. *Ophthalmology.* 113, 105–108 (2006).

[20] B. T. Kloss and R. Patel. Orbital compartment syndrome from retrobulbar hemorrhage. *Int. J. Emerg. Med.* 3, 521-522 (2010).

[21] V. Kratky, J. J. Hurwitz and D. R. Avram. Orbital compartment syndrome. Direct measurement of orbital tissue pressure: 1.Technique, *Can. J. Ophthalmol.* 25, 293–297 (1990).

[22] S. S. Hayreh, W. E. Kolder and T. A. Weingeist. Central retinal artery occlusion and retinal tolerance time. *Ophthalmology.* 87, 75–78 (1980).

[23] Y. Akar, K. C. Apaydin and A. Ozel. Acute orbital effects of retrobulbar injection on optic nerve head topography. *Br. J. Ophthalmol.* 88, 1573–1576 (2004).

[24] Ballard SR, Emergency lateral canthotomy and cantholysis: a simple procedure to preserve vision from sight threatening orbital hemorrhage, J Spec Oper Med. 2009 Summer; 9(3): 26-32.

[25] M. G. Yasargil. *Microneurosurgery, Volume I*, 1st edition. Thieme, pp215-224 (1984).

[26] E. Oester Jr, B. T. Fowler and J. C. Fleming. Inferior orbital septum release compared to lateral canthotomy and cantholysis in the management of orbital compartment syndrome. *Ophthal. Plast. Reconstr. Surg.* 28(1), 40–43 (2012).

[27] M. T. Sun, W. O. Chan and D. Selva. Traumatic orbital compartment syndrome: importance of lateral canthomy and cantholysis. *Emerg. Med. Australas*. 26(3), 274-278 (2014).

[28] M. Tso and R. L. Macdonald. Lateral canthotomy: part of a neurosurgeon's toolkit? *World Neurosurg*. 82(1–2), e189–e190 (2014).

Index

A

B

C

D

E

F

G

H

I

Q

R

S

T

U

V

W

Y

Z